Izabela Lopes Mendes

Physiotherapy in Uro-Gynecological and Breast Cancer

Izabela Lopes Mendes

Physiotherapy in Uro-Gynecological and Breast Cancer

Clinical Dysfunctions and Rehabilitation

ScienciaScripts

Imprint

Cover image: www.ingimage.com

This book is a translation from the original published under ISBN 978-613-9-62361-7.

Publisher:
Sciencia Scripts
is a trademark of
Dodo Books Indian Ocean Ltd. and OmniScriptum S.R.L publishing group

120 High Road, East Finchley, London, N2 9ED, United Kingdom
Str. Armeneasca 28/1, office 1, Chisinau MD-2012, Republic of Moldova, Europe
Printed at: see last page
ISBN: 978-620-7-72200-6

Summary

1. URO-GYNAECOLOGICAL CANCER

Overall, the most common types of cancer in the population are prostate cancer in men (68,000 cases) and breast cancer in women (60,000 cases) (MINISTÉRIO DA SAÙDE, 2018).

Gynecological cancer is currently considered a public health problem, characterized as a malignant neoplasm with a high incidence in women. In Brazil, estimates for 2018/2019 point to an incidence of 16,370 new cases of cervical cancer, 6,150 new cases of ovarian cancer and 6,600 new cases of cancer of the uterine body (MINISTÉRIO DA SAÙDE, 2018).

In the Southeast, the ten most common types of cancer are: breast cancer (30,880 cases), colon and rectum (10,600 cases), trachea, bronchus and lung (5,650 cases), cervix (4,420 cases), thyroid gland (4.330 cases), uterine body (3,400 cases), stomach (3,280 cases), ovary (2,850 cases), non-Hodgkin's lymphoma (2,530 cases) and central nervous system (2,450 cases) (MINISTÉRIO DA SAÙDE, 2018).

The elucidation of genetic mutations in the last century led to the discovery and understanding of hereditary syndromes associated with malignancies of the female genital tract. The discovery of the BRCA1 and BRCA2 genes in the early 1990s identified the main causative factor, in which women with mutations in these genes have an increased risk of developing breast carcinoma by 40-85%, and ovarian carcinoma by 10-39% (WONG; NGEOW, 2015).

Germline gene mutations play an important role in carcinogenesis (the process in which normal cells turn into cancer cells) due to DNA double strand breaks, chromosomal alteration, apoptosis and the cell cycle. The most lethal damage is DNA strand breaks, which are associated with ageing as a result of structural variations in the genome, cellular senescence and apoptosis, resulting in neurodegeneration, cancer, impaired regenerative capacity and inflammation (BEN-AHARON et al., 2018).

The evolution of gynaecological cancer is characterized by local invasion of the interstitial spaces of the pelvic connective tissue, and dissemination through the lymphatic system, which can reach other anatomical pathways, such as the vagina and bloodstream, and cause distant metastases and nerve compression (MARIN et al., 2014).

According to Chen et al. (2017), women with breast, uterine or ovarian cancer have a higher risk of developing a secondary cancer compared to the general population. This can be attributed, for example, in women with breast cancer, to estrogen receptor, tamoxifen use and reproductive risks, as well as BRCA 1 and BRCA 2 gene mutations in young women.

Ovarian cancer is considered the malignant neoplasm with the leading cause of death among gynecological neoplasms worldwide. Approximately 85 to 90% of malignant neoplasms are of the epithelial type, typically diagnosed in the late stages of the disease (ZHOU et al., 2015).

The main cause of death from ovarian cancer is the first unspecific symptoms of the disease, in which 70% of women are diagnosed at a late stage of the disease, when the tumor has already settled in the abdominal cavity, stage III and IV, with a survival rate of 15 to 29%, while 88% of women survive more than 5 years when diagnosed at stage I (HENTZE et al., 2017).

Ovarian cancer is described as a range of neoplasms with different histopathological characteristics, clinical evolution and response to treatment, which are grouped into two main types: type I and type II. Type I ovarian cancer has painless clinical features, low-grade carcinoma, with limitrophic and low-risk endometrioid. Type II ovarian cancer includes high-grade serous carcinoma, undifferentiated and carcinosarcoma, present in an advanced and highly aggressive stage (LUPIA; CAVALLARO, 2017).

Cervical cancer is one of the most common cancers among women in Brazil. Based on the evidence that persistent infection with carcinogenic human papillomavirus (HPV) types is the main cause, screening is carried out by cervical pap smear every 3 years in women aged 25 to 64, with the aim of identifying pre-invasive or invasive lesions at an early stage (KUPERMAN et al., 2015).

The main treatment for patients diagnosed with endometrial cancer and invasive cervical cancer is the surgical procedure of hysterectomy, with or without salpingo-oophorectomy, and pelvic lymphadenectomy, which remove the primary tumor and identify the risk of recurrence (BOGANI et al., 2015).

According to Choi et al. (2018) lymph node positivity and tumor mass size are significant prognostic factors in relation to recurrence and death in women with cervical cancer.

In cases of cervical cancer, the International Federation of Gynecology and Obstetrics (FIGO) recommends that patients with cancer at a stage that does not show evidence of tumor invasion into the lymphatic space (IA1), conservative therapy with cervical conization or simple hysterectomy is indicated. However, patients at risk of lymphatic spread (stage IA2 or IB1 cervical cancer) should be treated with radial hysterectomy and pelvic lymphadenectomy. Patients with more advanced stages (IB2 or IIA cervical cancer) should be treated with chemotherapy and radiotherapy, or combined therapy, and radical hysterectomy and pelvic lymphadenectomy (WARE; NAGELL, 2010).

High doses of irradiation to the pelvic lymph nodes contribute to late and serious complications in the genitourinary and gastrointestinal tracts. In many cases, pelvic lymph node dissection becomes an integral part of surgical treatment, and occurs in 7.1% of cases of ovarian cancer, 17.7% in uterine cancer, and 15.5% in cases of cervical cancer, which is considered a risk factor for the development of lymphedema due to the obstruction of lymph flow in the lower limbs (TADA et al., 2009; CHOI et al., 2018).

Therapeutic procedures for gynecological cancer can cause pelvic dysfunctions due to surgical trauma to the sympathetic, parasympathetic and somatic branches of the autonomic nervous system. According to the literature, after the surgical procedure, numerous factors can influence nerve damage, such as postoperative inflammation, local edema, transient nerve damage and decreased blood supply (ROH et al., 2015).

Marin et al. (2014) stated that early complications are intra-abdominal bleeding, supra-aponeurotic hematoma and genital fistulas. Late complications were voiding dysfunction, lower limb lymphedema, urethral stricture, incisional hernia, persistent pelvic pain, intestinal obstruction and sexual dysfunction.

According to the study by Pakbaz, Rolfsman and Lofgren (2017), women are not adequately informed before gynecological surgery. The results showed that 1 in 4 women undergoing hysterectomy received information about the possible effects of surgery on bladder and sexual function.

Urinary dysfunctions are the most frequent long-term complications after gynecological cancers, including symptoms such as sensory loss, bladder storage and partial emptying dysfunctions, urinary incontinence and detrusor muscle instability, which occur due to the sectioning of the nerves of the pelvic plexus during radical surgery (MARIN et al., 2014; ROH et al., 2015).

It is believed that surgery for gynecological cancers results in damage to the pelvic vascularization and innervation of the pelvic floor muscles, which causes damage to the urinary, anorectal and genital systems, as well as interfering with patients' quality of life (OSANN et al., 2014).

Many types of conventional radical surgery for gynecological cancers show 5-year survival rates in more than 90% of patients, however, they can cause urinary dysfunctions in 12% to 85%, such as bladder hypotonia and urinary incontinence, and colorectal dysfunctions, in which constipation occurs in 5% to 10% of women. Sexual dysfunctions are considerable after the surgical procedure, including decreased sexual interest, orgasm and vaginal dryness (KIM et al., 2015).

Hysterectomy is associated with short and long-term adverse changes, such as vaginal shortening, pelvic nerve damage, decreased sensitivity, vaginal lubrication, sexual desire, dyspareunia and early menopause (GILBERT; USSHER; PERZ, 2011).

According to Manchana (2011), voiding alterations are prevalent in gynecological cancer patients after radical hysterectomy, but do not influence the quality of life of patients when compared to the total abdominal hysterectomy technique.

Currently, modified radical hysterectomy has been proposed, as it aims to fully spare the plane of the autonomic nerve, in which the spontaneous return of urination varies between 8 and 14 days, compared to radical hysterectomy in which this return lasts for more than 20 days after surgery (WENWEN et al., 2014).

Yi et al. (2014) stated that the most prevalent postoperative complications, regardless of surgical technique, are bladder dysfunction, pelvic discomfort, ureterovaginal fistula, intestinal obstruction and thromboembolic disease.

Deep vein thrombosis and pulmonary embolism are important causes of postoperative mortality and morbidity in gynecological surgeries, with a high risk of developing deep vein thrombosis due to hypercoagulation, immobility and vascular injuries (ZHANG et al., 2015).

According to Chen et al. (2015) postoperative pain occurs due to a combination of factors, such as the physical damage caused by the surgical incision, inflammation, stimulation of visceral pain and nerve endings, which can inhibit mobility, and lead to other complications, such as deep vein thrombosis, pulmonary embolism and pneumonia. Patients with post-operative pain tend to be admitted to hospital with frequent readmissions, which leads to increased healthcare costs.

Kim et al. (2015) stated that urinary, anorectal and sexual dysfunctions are caused by damage to the pelvic autonomic nerves, which are responsible for the neurogenic control of urinary and rectal functions, and for providing blood supply to the female genital tract, which affects sexual activity due to a lack of lubrication.

Kanao et al. (2014) stated that the main cause of dysfunction is the injury to the pelvic plexus and its bladder branches that occurs after hysterectomy, which is responsible for triggering neurogenic bladder.

According to Marin et al. (2014) and Kato (2013), patients who do not experience the sensation of urinating, replace it with other perceptions, such as abdominal distension, tension in the pelvic region, discomfort, and over time associate it with a full bladder. In this way, they learn to empty their bladder over a period of time, and some patients need intermittent urinary catheters. Some symptoms are common in relation to bladder emptying deficiency, such as dysuria, bladder residue, overflow incontinence and recurrent urinary tract infections.

Li et al. (2018) stated that after radiotherapy the incidence of complications is high, late and difficult to estimate, with an average time of 10 months for the onset of radiation cystitis and 12 months for ureteral obstruction.

Urinary fistulas can occur as a result of injuries to the uterine wall, terminal ureter, vagina and pelvic tissue, in which the majority of cases are related to extensive dissection due to ischemic damage or radiotherapy. The incidence of urinary fistulas after hysterectomy is reported at 0.14 to 20%, and 0.6 to 5.1% in women after cervical cancer. Urological fistula causes constant leakage of urine, which significantly increases postoperative morbidity (KARKHANIS; PATEL; GALAAL, 2012; URH et al., 2013).

Vesico-cutaneous fistula results in leakage of urine from the bladder to the surface, caused by iatrogenic injury, trauma, radical pelvic surgery and irradiation of malignancies, which results in discomfort and disability of the patient (KIM et al., 2018).

Another very common complication is pelvic organ prolapse, defined as the displacement of pelvic organs from the inside to the outside of the vaginal canal, described as prolapse of the anterior, posterior and apical compartments of the vagina. The complaint first reported by women is the feeling of heaviness in the vaginal canal, followed by increased urinary frequency, urgency, incontinence, intermittent flow, feeling of incomplete emptying, constipation and the need for vaginal touch to reposition the organ in more advanced stages (OZENGIN et al., 2017).

With regard to colorectal dysfunctions, the symptoms most often cited in the literature were chronic constipation, anal incontinence or gas, and difficulty or loss of desire for bowel movements.

Altered anorectal function often occurs post-radiation, associated with high rates of diarrhea and frequent bowel movements, suggesting that acute and daily toxicity during radiation therapy increases severe late toxicity, which affects quality of life. In patients with chronic or intermittent diarrhea, it is possible to notice impaired absorption of bile acids and increased proliferation of bacteria. In addition, damage to the external anal sphincter muscle, reduced rectal capacity and impaired sensory functions are considered important factors contributing to anal motor dysfunction (NORONHA et al., 2013).

Khoshbaten et al. (2011) confirmed the diagnosis of irritable bowel syndrome in 8% of women after hysterectomy, in which, along with abdominal pain, symptoms such as chronic constipation and abnormal bowel movements, and less prevalent symptoms such as diarrhea and mucus elimination, were reported.

Sexual problems are commonly reported among women after gynecological cancer, such as a shortened vagina, involuntary contraction of the vagina, decreased lubrication, dyspareunia, bleeding, loss of pleasure, desire and sexual satisfaction, factors that are aggravated after radiotherapy (BAKKER et al., 2014).

Dyspareunia, vaginal dryness and difficulties in achieving orgasm are considered common post-operative side effects. Vaginal dryness is related to lower levels of estrogen after ovarian resection (bilateral oophorectomy), as without this hormone the vaginal lining becomes thinner and loses its elasticity, causing vaginal atrophy, which contributes to pain during intercourse and decreased libido. The lack of vaginal and clitoral sensitivity, which occurs mainly due to damage to the nerves involved in arousal, leads to a decrease in orgasmic response (MARIN et al., 2014).

Goktas et al. (2015) stated that during cervical ablation surgery, the hypogastric plexus, which is responsible for sympathetic innervation of the pelvic region, can be damaged. In addition, the removal of the uterus generates a feeling of inability to reproduce and anxiety about sexual activity, which has a negative impact on social life and communication with the partner, and contributes to increased levels of depression.

According to Levin et al. (2010) women with a history of depressive illnesses show less arousal, physical pleasure and emotional satisfaction with their partner, in which declining mental health can be considered a risk factor for the development of sexual dysfunction.

Studies have reported that sexual response is diminished due to hormonal changes, ovarian androgen, and anatomical changes, removal of the cervix, as well as psychological factors, in which depression has a negative effect on postoperative symptoms and aspects of sexual activity (KOMISARUK; FRANGOS; WHIPPLE, 2011; CARTER et al., 2012).

Grover et al. (2012) stated that the most common late effects reported by patients diagnosed with gynecological malignancies were cognitive, sexual and intestinal alterations, peripheral neuropathy and skin color. The findings of the study show that women with cervical cancer present with scarring in the bladder region and loss of flexibility, associated with changes in cognitive function, sexual dysfunction and peripheral neuropathy, while in women with uterine cancer these symptoms are associated with intestinal changes. However, in women with ovarian cancer, cognitive, gastrointestinal, sexual and peripheral neuropathy alterations predominated.

Therefore, the risk of pelvic injury is inherent in the surgical treatment of gynecological cancers, which results in the need for information for women, so that they can better understand their health conditions and be monitored by the health team in the short and long term.

1.1 VOIDING DYSFUNCTION IN WOMEN

The female pelvic floor is closely connected between the pelvic bones, muscles, fasciae and ligaments. Structurally, the support system for the pelvic organs is carried out by the group of muscles that lift the anus and are suspended by the endopelvic fascia. During rest, the integral connective tissue has the function of maintaining the pelvic organs for the storage of urine and feces, and consequently relaxes according to demand to allow mobility of the organ for excretion (BHATTARAI; STAAT, 2017).

The muscles of the pelvic floor are composed of approximately 70% type I fibers, called slow contraction fibers, responsible for supporting the pelvic organs, and 30% type II fibers, called fast contraction fibers, responsible for urethral closure in activities that cause increased intra-abdominal pressure, facts that are extremely important for the continence mechanism (MARTINHO et al., 2015).

As the resting tone of the pelvic muscles decreases, ligament laxity sets in, causing an anatomical distortion that leads to an attenuation of contraction capacity and malfunction. This mechanism becomes harmful due to the avulsion of the pelvic muscle or the rupture of the connective tissue (LUCENTE et al., 2017).

However, pelvic injuries damage muscle contraction and lead to pelvic floor dysfunction, such as incontinence, pelvic organ prolapse and sexual dysfunction (BHATTARAI; STAAT, 2017).

Urinary incontinence is a medical condition with a negative impact on quality of life, as well as imposing an economic burden on the health system and society. Urinary incontinence occurs regardless of age group, racial and ethnic groups, where the prevalence remains between 2 and 4 times higher in women when compared to men, with stress urinary incontinence being prevalent in 50% of women with complaints of urinary loss (VILSBOLL et al., 2018).

According to the International Urogynecological Association (IUGA), urinary incontinence is defined as the involuntary loss of urine and there are two main subtypes: stress incontinence and urge incontinence. Stress incontinence is the complaint of urine loss associated with coughing, sneezing or physical exertion due to increased intra-abdominal pressure, while urge incontinence is defined as urine loss associated with the sudden urge to delay urination. However, when these two subtypes are associated, it is called mixed urinary incontinence (AOKI et al., 2018).

UUI is defined as urinary leakage preceded by an imminent urge to urinate and is usually associated with overactive bladder syndrome. This urinary urgency is characterized by polaciuria and nocturia in the absence of urine infection or other conditions, which can be associated with neurological or idiopathic injury, however the literature is still scarce as to the pathophysiological mechanism. Hypotheses suggest four mechanisms of idiopathic detrusor overactivity, such as: alteration of the micturition reflex mechanism, attenuation of bladder innervation, release of acetylcholine in the parasympathetic plate during filling and activation of urothelial receptors (MOTA, 2017).

Stress urinary incontinence has been described by two mechanisms: urethral hypermobility due to loss of support of the bladder neck and urethra, as well as intrinsic sphincter deficiency, weakness of the urinary sphincter itself (MARQUES, SILVA; AMARAL, 2011).

According to Torre and Miller (2017) the main risk factors involved in the development of SUI include pregnancy, childbirth, hysterectomy, obesity, age and family history.

The prevalence of lower urinary tract dysfunction is common after hysterectomy (70-85%), with stress urinary incontinence accounting for 40% of cases (HEYDARI; MOTAGHED, ABBASZADEH, 2017).

According to the aforementioned authors, urodynamics plays an important role in understanding and quantifying the severity of SUI. Severity assessment can be measured by the valsalva leak point pressure (VLPP), which indicates the pressure needed to overcome the bladder's resistance to increased intra-abdominal pressure during exertion, in which values below 60 cmH2O are indicative of severe SUI, while values between 60 and 90 cmH2O are considered intermediate grade, and above 90 cmH2O as low grade.

Treatment resources for SUI include physiotherapy with conservative techniques such as pelvic muscle training, *biofeedback* and electrostimulation, and surgical treatment which aims to functionally correct the urinary sphincter and urethra by injecting submucosal polymers around the sphincter, slings, among others (MOTA, 2017).

1.2 SEXUAL DYSFUNCTION IN WOMEN

The decrease in sexual desire can be attributed to numerous factors, including biological, psychological and social variables. Currently, it is believed that sexual desire is regulated by neurotransmitters and hormones from excitatory pathways, such as dopamine, norepinephrine, oxytocin, and inhibitory pathways, such as serotonin and opioids, in which decreased neural activation and lack of disinhibition impair vasocongestion, vaginal lubrication and orgasm (CLAYTON et al., 2018).

Urinary incontinence negatively influences a woman's sex life, triggering problems such as loss of urine during intercourse, nocturnal urinary leakage related to urgency or fear and insecurity due to stench, which causes a change in the woman's image and self-esteem (MOTA, 2017).

According to the International Association of Urogynecology and the International Continence Society, coital incontinence is characterized as a complaint of involuntary loss of urine during coitus, a common symptom that negatively affects the quality of life of sexually active women (LAU; HUANG; SU, 2017).

The pathogenesis is still unknown, however it is associated that incontinence of coitus is more prevalent in women with SUI during the act of penetration, and incontinence during orgasm due to detrusor overactivity. However, both cause a reduction in sexual desire and the ability to reach orgasm (LAU; HUANG; SU, 2017).

Radiotherapy for gynecological cancer leads to ovarian insufficiency, with a consequent decrease in estradiol and progesterone levels, early menopause and loss of libido, as well as damage to the vaginal epithelium, vascular structures and connective tissue.

As a result, these changes cause vaginal obstruction and loss of elasticity, with consequent pain, bleeding and difficulty in sexual intercourse.

The literature reports that female sexual dysfunctions such as dyspareunia and vaginismus are characterized by difficulty in vaginal penetration during sexual intercourse; genito-pelvic pain or pain during vaginal penetration; fear and anxiety associated with penetration or pain; or compression of the pelvic muscles during attempted vaginal penetration (ZARSKI; BERKING; EBERT, 2018).

Physiotherapeutic intervention in women with vaginismus or dyspareunia includes pain management strategies, desensitization, pelvic floor exercises with a focus on teaching pelvic muscle relaxation.

Guner et al. (2018) conducted a descriptive study with the aim of examining the sexual functions of patients after gynecological surgery and brachytherapy. The results showed that most of the patients had sexual dysfunctions, and the authors emphasized that these women should be routinely evaluated for sexual dysfunctions, informed and advised about their sex life together with their partner.

Dyspareunia associated with anxiety contributes to reduced sexual intercourse, sexual desire and arousal (LIMA et al., 2018).

Mohktar et al. (2013) stated that among the many factors involved in sexual dysfunction, PFM function plays an important role. The muscles of the pelvic floor are crucial for genital arousal and achieving orgasm in women; however, weakness of the PFM provides inadequate arousal, which makes it difficult to achieve orgasm. Approximately 25 to 50% of women with decreased pelvic floor muscle function have sexual dysfunction.

1.3 . PHYSIOTHERAPEUTIC EVALUATION OF THE FEMALE PELVIC FLOOR

This topic highlights the importance of physiotherapy in the prevention, diagnosis and treatment of pelvic floor dysfunctions, using critical assessment criteria and specific therapeutic resources.

Figure 1 summarizes and proposes a sequence for physiotherapeutic assessment based on clinical evidence in pelvic dysfunctions.

Figure 1: Diagram of physiotherapeutic assessment in urogynecology.

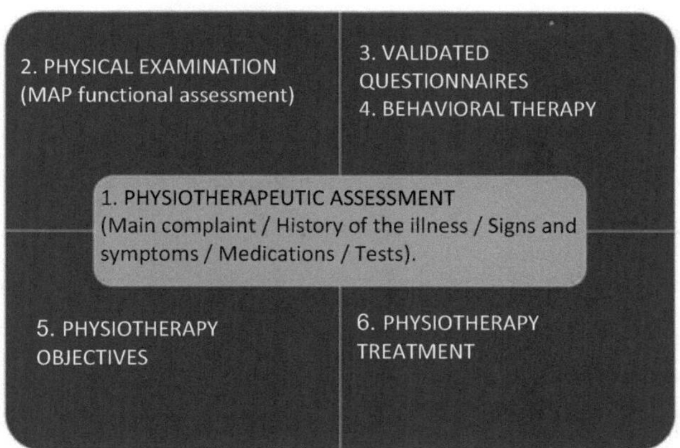

Source: author.

The physical assessment of patients with pelvic floor dysfunction includes a functional assessment of the pelvic floor, pelvic mobility, abdominal examination to assess the presence of pelvic masses, palpable bladder, tenderness, vaginal atrophy and dermatitis associated with incontinence.

The function of the pelvic floor muscles can be assessed using bidigital touch, visual observation, electromyography, ultrasound and magnetic resonance imaging. Physiotherapists commonly use bidigital touch to assess PFM function (SARTORI et al., 2015).

Manual palpation was first described by Kegel as a method of assessing the pelvic floor muscles. It is currently considered essential in assessing PFM function to quantify muscle strength and endurance, providing information on the severity of muscle weakness and the basis for planning physiotherapy treatment (CHEVALIER et al., 2014).

Functional assessment of the pelvic floor muscles is important for investigating muscle response, resting tone, quantifying strength, endurance, speed of contraction, ability to repeat and perform fast and slow contractions.

The most commonly used scales for assessing the pelvic floor musculature by two-digital touch are the Oxford Scale and the Perfect Scale (Power, Endurance, Repetition, Fast, Elevation, Co-contration and Timing) (TOSUN et al., 2016).

The digital touch quantitatively and qualitatively assesses the voluntary contraction of the pelvic floor muscles. To quantify the strength of the PFM, the therapist performs the vaginal touch with the first two phalanges of the second and third fingers smeared with lubricating gel and wearing gloves, then the therapist asks for maximum voluntary contraction, and may ask the patient to say the following command: "squeeze my fingers", the command to the patient is to contract the muscles as much as possible.

Therefore, strength can be classified according to the modified Oxford Scale as: 0 (nil), 1 (shaky), 2 (weak), 3 (moderate muscle contraction), 4 (good muscle contraction) to 5 (strong contraction) (ANGELO *et al.*, 2017).

To perform the PFM assessment, the patient can remain in the gynecological position (supine position) with her knees bent, hips flexed and abducted. She should be instructed on the correct way to contract the PFM, without co-contracting the abdominal muscles, adductors and glutes.

One of the perineal rehabilitation protocols at Clinica Spazio Saùde recommends that the physical examination be carried out with a full functional assessment of the pelvic floor muscles, as described below.

- Inspection: check for scars, color, hyperemia, edema and dystopia.
- Visual functional assessment: voluntary contraction, involuntary contraction and consequent relaxation of the PFM.

- Perineal palpation: adhesions, tenderness, painful points and muscle trophism.
- Bidigital touch in the vaginal canal to palpate basal tone and apply the Perfect Scale.

At the end of the clinical-functional assessment, validated questionnaires are used to subjectively measure the impact of sexual dysfunction and urinary incontinence on the patient's quality of life, such as the *King's Health Quaestinnaire*.

This is followed by additional guidance for the patient on the pathology and anatomy, using images that represent the pelvic floor.

The patient is also instructed in the importance of behavioral therapy, including home guidance on water intake habits, interval urination and filling out a voiding diary.

At the end of the first physiotherapy session, the patient is informed of the therapeutic objectives, which are clearly explained so that she can better understand the role and importance of physiotherapy treatment, as well as the use of invasive and non-invasive therapeutic techniques.

1.4 PHYSIOTHERAPEUTIC TREATMENT

Understanding the anatomy and contractility of the PFM is important for pelvic floor function, especially understanding tone and correct contraction, mechanisms that prevent pelvic organ prolapse and are responsible for continence (VOLLOYHAUG et al., 2016).

The physiotherapeutic approach is another standard in the first-line treatment of urinary and fecal incontinence, with emphasis on education about contraction and training of the pelvic floor muscles.

The training of the pelvic floor muscles was described in 1948 by Kegel and colleagues, who reported an improvement rate of 84% in different cases of urinary incontinence, and is considered as effective as conservative treatment (KASHANIAN et al., 2011).

Training of the pelvic floor muscles emerged more than 50 years ago, and to this day is considered effective in the treatment of urinary incontinence and is recommended as the first line of treatment for women with stress urinary incontinence, according to guidelines from the *European Association of Urology and the Japanese Urological Association* (FUJISAKI et al., 2018).

The therapist's verbal command is crucial for the proper performance of the contraction, which should guide the woman to contract the pelvic floor muscles before and during activities that cause increased intra-abdominal pressure, called "the Knack" (ANDRADE *et al.*, 2018).

Fujisaki et al. (2018) stated that it is essential for patients with SUI to learn how to correctly contract the pelvic floor muscles with PFM training programs, effectively contributing to the improvement of complaints.

The International Continence Society states that correct muscle contraction of the pelvic floor should result in ventral and cranial movement of the perineum, and upward movement of the pelvic organs, associated with anterior movement caused by the vaginal and rectal parts of the levators ani, i.e. internal lifting and tightening around the urethra, vagina and anus (SALMON *et al.*, 2017).

The levator ani muscles play an important role in the urinary and fecal continence mechanism, because when activated, their resulting force in the ventrecephalic direction compresses the rectum, vagina and urethra, which promotes urethrovesical elevation, together with ligaments, they act to support the pelvic organs (AMORIM et al., 2017).

Strengthening the pelvic floor muscles aims to improve the structural support of the pelvis, increasing hypertrophy of the pelvic muscles and connective tissues, promoting efficient activation of the motor unit, i.e. neural adaptation and preventing pelvic organ prolapse (OZENGIN; YILDIRIM; DURAN, 2015).

Maxwell et al. (2017) stated that the regular practice of repetitive muscle contractions of the pelvic floor generates a training effect on the musculature, increasing muscle strength and volume, structural support, endurance, normalizes resting tone, fiber recruitment and cognitive awareness in relation to body posture.

However, some points are relevant for gaining strength and muscular endurance, for example: overload, which can result in fatigue; specificity, in which the PFM should be trained in the activity that is close to the functional movement; maintenance and reversibility, i.e. they should be performed regularly (MAXWELL et al., 2017).

Another method cited in the literature is increasing PFM strength associated with training the transverse abdominis muscle (OZENGIN; YILDIRIM; DURAN, 2015).

The transverse abdominal muscle plays an important role in the continence mechanism, due to the fact that contraction of the transverse muscle facilitates tensioning of the pubococcygeus muscle of the levator ani (URQUHART et al., 2005; RAJKOWSKA-LABON et al., 2014).

According to Amorim et al. (2017) muscles around the hip, such as the obturator internus, also contribute to the continence mechanism and sexual function. The obturator internus has the function of abducting and externally rotating the hip, especially when flexed and in isometric tasks, in which its fascia is attached to the iliococcygeus portion of the levator ani by the arcus tendineus fascia pelvis.

The aforementioned authors defend the hypothesis of the combined action of PFM and the isometric force of hip abduction, due to the fact that intravaginal force is generated and maintained, however, they rule out the combined action of hip adduction because there are no anatomical and mechanical correlations between the hip adductor muscles (AMORIM et al., 2017).

The authors Cook et al. (2017) defend the hypothesis that aging has a deleterious effect on muscle mechanics, generating a decrease in force production and fibrosis of the obturator internus muscle.

In the first perineal rehabilitation sessions at Clinica Spazio Saùde, women with urinary incontinence are informed and instructed on the importance of correct PFM contraction.

The importance of concentration during the exercises is emphasized to these women, so that they focus their attention during the contraction of the PFM, isolating the contraction of accessory muscles, such as the abdominal muscles, hip adductors, glutes, among others.

However, when women report great difficulty in contracting the PFM or are unable to activate the muscles, the bidigital touch test is used to provide feedback for proper contraction.

According to Ong et al. (2015) approximately 30% of women are unable to perform isolated contractions of the pelvic floor with the help of written or verbal instructions, making it necessary to use biofeedback in order to improve muscle function and the execution of pelvic exercises.

The use of biofeedback associated with pelvic floor exercises requires the active participation of the patient, specialized equipment for converting physiological signals into visual and/or auditory signals and a trained professional (SANTOS et al., 2018).

The applicability of electromyographic biofeedback as visual feedback during PFM training can be considered a valuable therapeutic resource. It is defined as a non-invasive technique that analyzes the electrical potentials generated by muscle fibers during contraction, with the aim of providing the patient with learning the correct PFM contraction, as well as muscle awareness and activation (HILL; ALAPPATTU, 2017).

PFM training with the help of electromyographic biofeedback is carried out using an intravaginal probe, which is more precise and objective for assessing muscle activation, or by placing surface electrodes on the external anal sphincter, both of which provide visualization of the signal amplitude for analysis of resting tone and contraction and relaxation cycles (HILL; ALAPPATTU,

2017).

The applicability of electrostimulation in the treatment of urinary symptoms emerged in the early 1960s, but it wasn't until 1963 that Caldwell presented the first clinical study of electrostimulation for the control of urinary complaints. Moore then reapplied the study, showing improvement in 10 out of 18 patients with urinary incontinence. In 1989, Tanagho and colleagues carried out a study on electrical modulation by implanting an electrode in the ventral roots of S3 and S4 in patients with voiding disorders (ABELLO; DAS, 2018).

Sacral neuromodulation has an effect on spinal afferents, sympathetic and parasympathetic preganglionic afferents. The S3 nerve root is of extreme clinical relevance in patients with micturition dysfunction, as it consists of sensory fibers from the pelvic floor and parasympathetic fibers from the detrusor, in which synapses and connections travel to the CNS via ascending and descending spinal pathways until they reach the brainstem and the brain centers of bladder control, such as the micturition pontine center, in response, the final effect on the modulation of reflex pathways.

Currently, electrical stimulation has been used to treat bladder disorders such as urinary retention and incontinence. The most commonly used modalities are transcutaneous electrical stimulation (TENS), percutaneous tibial nerve stimulation and sacral neuromodulation (SUN et al., 2017).

Transcutaneous Electrical Stimulation (TENS) is a non-invasive technique, easy to apply and low cost compared to other modalities, which stimulates the sensory fibers of the pudendal nerve at low frequencies of 2 to 5Hz, which alters the electrical impulses of the nerve fibers promoting improvement in blood circulation of the pelvic organs, bladder sensitivity and detrusor contractility (SUN et al., 2017).

Schmitt et al. (2017) stated that the electrical pulses stimulate afferents from the pudendal nerve, which consequently activate contraction efferents from the striated muscles of the pelvis and generate inhibition of detrusor hyperactivity.

Thiele massage is an effective technique for treating dyspareunia due to the sensitivity of the pelvic floor muscles (SILVA et al., 2017).

It's a simple technique that can be taught to women to perform at home. After positioning the index finger in the vaginal canal, the woman is instructed to perform oscillatory and rhythmic movements in a "U" shape, upwards, laterally and downwards, the frequency and duration of which must be determined by the physiotherapist.

Vaginal dilators are therapeutic devices with a smooth, cylindrical shape that increase in diameter according to the woman's condition and level of adherence to therapy. The use of vaginal dilators is recommended for women who have undergone pelvic radiotherapy or those who report pain and discomfort during sexual intercourse. They are often indicated to prevent and minimize vaginal stenosis and scarring, adhesions, relaxation of the pelvic floor muscles and pain relief (LEE, 2018).

Studies recommend the use of vaginal dilators between 2 and 4 weeks after the end of radiotherapy, or when the vaginal mucosa has healed, usually around 4 weeks, which can be used 2 to 3 times a week and reduced if the patient resumes sexual intercourse (BAKKER *et al.*, 2014).

It is important to advise the patient on the gradual use of the cylinder circumference, as well as the time of use, which according to the literature ranges from 5 to 10 minutes (BAKKER *et al.*, 2014).

The vaginal pessary is a device that has been used for centuries in the conservative treatment of pelvic organ prolapse and incontinence. Incontinence pessaries are silicone or rubber devices positioned transvaginally to promote the urethrovesical junction with the same purpose as the surgical vaginal sling implant (AL-SHAIKH et al., 2018).

The purpose of the brace is to support the urethra and bladder wall by providing gentle compression of the urethra against the pubic bone, in order to prevent urine leakage when intra-abdominal pressure increases (AL-SHAIKH et al., 2018).

Different types are available on the market, including the ring device with support, characterized by easy insertion, the incontinence plate device, characterized by easy insertion and removal, which are commonly used in patients with SUI, and the Uresta device. These have the function of stabilizing the urethra and increasing urethral resistance (AL-SHAIKH et al., 2018).

The use of pessaries is a good therapeutic option for urinary incontinence in women of any age, with the advantages of being minimally invasive, immediate relief of symptoms and low cost (AL-SHAIKH et al., 2018).

2. BREAST CANCER

Breast cancer is currently a public health problem, considered the leading cause of death from malignant cancer in the female population, with an estimated 59,700 new cases of breast cancer in Brazil in 2018/2019, an estimated 56.3 cases per 100,000 women (MINISTÉRIO DA SAÙDE, 2018).

According to the José Alencar Gomes da Silva National Cancer Institute (INCA), in 2008 there were an estimated 36 million deaths due to Non-Communicable Diseases (NCDs), responsible for the illness and death of the population worldwide, with a prevalence of 48% due to cardiovascular diseases and 21% due to cancer (MINISTÉRIO DA SAÙDE, 2015; MINISTÉRIO DA SAÙDE, 2018).

The incidence by geographic region shows that breast cancer is more frequent in the South (73.07/100,000) and Southeast (69.50/100,000), representing 70% of the occurrence of new cases, followed by the Midwest (51.96/100,000) and Northeast (40.36/100,000), however, in the North breast cancer is the second most incident tumor (19.21/100,000), with cervical cancer prevailing (MINISTÉRIO DA SAÙDE, 2018).

Human breast carcinogenesis is a complex process involving a large number of genetic mutations that normally occur in epithelial cells. It is characterized by the disordered growth of mutated cells, resulting from alterations in specific sectors of the genetic code, with an increase in proliferation and a decrease in cell apoptosis, which alters the phenotype of normal tissue. The development of the tumor mass is slow or rapidly progressive, depending on the speed of cell duplication, with varied clinical and morphological manifestations (MACON; FENTON, 2013; MARGAN et al., 2016).

Breast cancer encompasses heterogeneous phenotypes with different anatomopathological characteristics, which are subclassified according to histological type and grade, estrogen receptor (ER), progesterone receptor (PR) and human epidermal growth factor (HER-2 / Human Epidermal Growth Factor Receptor - type 2) (LESURF et al., 2016).

According to the study by Lobbezoo et al. (2016), the two main histological subtypes of breast cancer are invasive ductal carcinoma (IDC) and invasive lobular carcinoma (ILC). Patients with ILC are older at the time of diagnosis of primary breast cancer, with a higher rate of initial bone metastasis (46.5% versus 34.8% for IDC) and fewer metastatic sites compared to IDC (23.7% versus 30.9%), with an overall survival of 29 months for patients with ILC and 25 months for patients with IDC.

Ductal carcinoma of the breast, also known as invasive ductal carcinoma or ductal carcinoma not otherwise specified (NOS), accounts for around 70% to 80% of breast cancer cases, characterized by a high frequency of axillary lymph node involvement and a worse prognosis. Invasive lobular carcinoma accounts for 10% to 15% of breast cancers, while other histological types with a more favorable prognosis are rarer, such as medullary carcinoma (5% to 7%), tubular carcinoma (1% to 3%) and mucinous carcinoma (2%) (STEIN et al., 2016).

Inflammatory breast cancer is rare with an incidence of 1% to 5% of all breast carcinomas, with more aggressive histological features and poor survival. Clinically, inflammatory breast cancer is characterized by redness, heat, swelling and an orange peel appearance on the skin, all of which involve at least a third of the breast. The average age at diagnosis is 52 years, compared to 57 years for other types of breast cancer (MOSLEHI et al., 2016).

The etiology of breast cancer is multifactorial, and several factors are related to the risk of developing the disease, such as the interaction of genetic factors, age, reproductive history and bad habits or lifestyle (sedentary lifestyle, smoking, alcoholism, obesity) (BRENNER et al., 2016; PARSA et al., 2016).

Progesterone and estrogen affect the cell cycle and alter the progression of cancer. High levels of estrogen are implicated in breast carcinogenesis, as binding to the estradiol receptor induces the synthesis and stimulates the secretion of growth factors, which induces cell division (STEIN et al., 2016). For this reason, women with early menarche, late menopause, hormone replacement therapy, fewer pregnancies and those who have not breastfed are at greater risk of developing breast cancer (PARSA et al., 2016).

Obesity and a sedentary lifestyle are factors that increase the risk of developing breast cancer in older women and contribute to progression at all ages, mainly due to changes in the insulin resistance pathway (BRENNER et al., 2016).

On the other hand, the substances in cigarette smoke can cause alterations in the transcription mechanism that regulates the expression of genes involved in the transformation of healthy epithelial cells, as well as the proliferation of epithelial tumor cells in the mammary gland (PÉREZ-SOLIS et al., 2016).

Excessive alcohol consumption is one of the bad habits that contribute to the etiology of breast cancer. In addition to promoting carcinogenesis, alcohol stimulates the migration and invasion of cells overexpressing the ErbB2 receptor (an oncogene located on chromosome 17 that is expressed in 20% to 30% of breast cancer cases), increases the aggressiveness of breast cancer cells and the risk of metastasis and recurrence (XU et al., 2016).

The elucidation of genetic mutations in the last century led to the discovery and understanding of hereditary syndromes associated with tumors. The discovery of the BRCA1 and BRCA2 genes (Breast Cancer type 1 and 2) at the beginning of the 1990s identified the main cause, in which women with mutations in these genes have an increased risk of developing breast carcinoma of 47% to 66% and 40% to 57% respectively, at the age of 40 to 50 years, and sporadically at the age of 60 to 70 years (WONG; NGEOW, 2015; MAESHIMA et al., 2016).

Age is the most important demographic risk factor for the development of cancers, including breast cancer. The risk of developing breast cancer is higher in old age, due to exposure to carcinogens over time and the decrease in the strength of the immune system (PARSA et al., 2016).

According to Brenner et al. (2016), the average age for developing breast cancer is 55 years old, where the incidence increases exponentially until the age of 40, and linearly with age. However, younger women tend to have fewer comorbidities and better tolerance to treatment toxicity, but are treated more aggressively due to the severity of the disease.

Breast cancer screening aims to reduce mortality and morbidities related to advanced stages of the disease (PROVENCHER et al., 2016). Mammography screening is essential for the early detection of breast cancer, capable of detecting the disease at an early stage and reducing mortality by 15% to 25% (LOPES et al., 2016).

Breast cancer treatment is initiated after assessing the clinical stage and histological type of the tumor, which are decisive factors in choosing the type of surgical procedure, conservative or non-conservative (TOVAR; ZANDONADE; AMORIM, 2014).

In 1894, William Halsted performed the surgery named after him, the Halsted radical mastectomy, which involved large incisions and extensive tissue ablation, such as the mammary gland, both pectoral muscles and all the axillary tissue. However, the extent of the resection led to significant morbidities such as paresthesia, lymphedema and pneumothorax. For this reason, the hypothesis of the uselessness of the intervention arose in 1935 by Haagensen, and was confirmed in 1971 by Bernard Fisher, after the publication of a controlled study comparing the Halsted mastectomy technique to modified radical mastectomy. At the time, David H. Patey modified Halsted's surgery by preserving the pectoral muscle. In 1972, the current standard was created, the modified radical mastectomy by John Madden, with the aim of preserving one or both pectoral muscles (PLESCA *et al.*, 2016).

Questions are frequently asked about prophylactic mastectomy, especially among women who fear the recurrence of the disease. Removal of the contralateral breast is a radical and irreversible prophylactic alternative that is effective in reducing the risk of developing contralateral breast cancer, but there is insufficient evidence that it improves survival (YAKOUB *et al.*, 2015).

Conservative surgery, considered the procedure of choice in the initial phase of breast cancer, includes the removal of the tumor involving a safety margin of healthy tissue. In this intervention, breast tissue is preserved and it can be performed using the quadrantectomy (segmental resection) or tumorectomy (removal of the tumor with a margin of breast tissue free of neoplasia around it) techniques (TOVAR; ZANDONADE; AMORIM, 2014).

The status of the axillary lymph node is considered a prognostic and determining factor in the treatment of breast cancer, which must be associated with the biological characteristics of the primary tumor and subsequent adjuvant treatment (ALSAIF *et al.*, 2015).

The sentinel lymph node is the first lymph node within the lymphatic network to receive lymph drainage from a tumor, and the first site of metastasis. Sentinel lymph node biopsy is a minimally invasive procedure that was introduced in the early 1990s and has now become the standard for axillary staging. Clinically, sentinel lymph node biopsy involves the local removal of axillary lymph nodes (level I) by staining the tissue with blue dye (ALSAIF *et al.*, 2015; HAN; YANG; ZUO, 2016; YEN *et al., 2016*).

Dissection of positive lymph nodes or complete or partial axillary lymphadenectomy is performed in order to clinically stage the disease and achieve local control by removing axillary nodes, with the aim of reducing the risk of lymphatic metastasis (SMEETS *et al.*, 2013).

Axillary dissection is currently the standard treatment for patients with metastatic axillary lymph nodes; however, it has a high incidence of lymphedema, ranging from 6% to 57%. On the other hand, in patients with a negative axilla, sentinel lymph node biopsy is recommended and reduces morbidities such as lymphedema, but the incidence remains significant, averaging 13% of cases (HAN *et al.*, 2016).

Both surgical techniques, conservative or non-conservative, are commonly accompanied by axillary lymph node dissection, as they are common sites of metastasis and an important prognostic indicator, in which survival rates are similar (HWANG *et al.*, 2013; CHENG et *al.*, 2016).

The therapeutic modalities for breast cancer involve both radiotherapy and hormone therapy to reduce the risk of local-regional recurrence, as well as chemotherapy for systemic treatment, and can be used in the neoadjuvant, adjuvant and palliative contexts. Studies have shown the benefits of chemotherapy for reducing tumor mass, which is widely used in cases of women with locally advanced cancer and a high risk of recurrence (ADEMUYIWA; ELLIS; MA, 2013).

Radiotherapy is applied with the aim of reducing tumor size before surgery or destroying remaining cells after surgery. In women at an early stage of cancer, with indications for breast-conserving surgery, radiotherapy is considered the gold standard for reducing the risk of local recurrence (JERZAK *et al.*, 2017).

Rief *et al.* (2017) stated that preoperative radiotherapy followed by mastectomy provided good long-term loco-regional control in the study in question, with control rates of 91% at 10 years, 89% at 20 years and 89% at 30 years.

Adjuvant hormone therapy with the use of selective estrogen receptor modulators, such as tamoxifen or toremifene, is considered standard endocrine therapy because it reduces the risk of annual recurrence by 50% and the mortality rate by 31% after diagnosis. Both are responsible for inducing apoptosis and inhibiting hormonal stimulation of breast cancer cell proliferation (BHATTA, 2013; QUIN *et al., 2013*).

According to Li *et al.* (2016) endocrine therapy is a widely used strategy after breast cancer, however, adverse symptoms are often reported by women that interfere with daily activities and decrease the quality of life of breast cancer survivors, such as a sudden episode of internal heat sensation, often followed by chills, redness in the face and upper body, accompanied by deep sweating and dizziness.

Clinical complications are common after breast cancer surgery. In addition to the long-term risk of developing lymphedema, numerous acute complications can occur, such as hemorrhage, tissue necrosis, wound infection and seromas, which represent the most frequent post-surgical complication (CHENG *et al.*, 2016).

According to the study by Samuel *et al.* (2015), the primary consequences of cancer treatment reported by women are fatigue, anxiety, depression, loss of appetite, decreased joint range, pain, sedentary lifestyle and intolerance to physical exercise.

Other symptoms that contribute to the limitation of shoulder joint range are common after breast cancer surgery, such as disuse, pain, numbness and decreased strength, which begin within a few days of surgery and tend to increase over time. In the second week after surgery, 40% of patients show a reduction in shoulder abduction movement, 37% show a reduction in flexion movement and 17% to 33% a reduction in muscle strength. Decreased shoulder joint range and muscle strength are problems reported up to four years after surgery, and can contribute to the development of lymphedema (MORONE *et al.*, 2014; GRITSENKO *et al.*, 2015).

Post-mastectomy pain syndrome is defined as chronic neuropathic pain after any type of breast surgery, with moderate intensity and neuropathic characteristics present in the ipsilateral breast and upper limb, lasting more than 6 months. According to the literature, the clinical picture occurs due to nerve damage during surgery, such as the intercostobrachial, medial pectoral, lateral pectoral, long thoracic and thoracodorsal nerves (BEYAZ *et al.*, 2016; BRACKSTONE *et al.*, 2016; LARSSON; SORENSEN; BILLE, 2017).

Lymphedema is defined as chronic and progressive swelling of the ipsilateral limb, which arises due to mechanisms such as the surgical removal of lymphatic structures, which impair the transport of lymph; surgical scars that occlude the lymphatic vessels or generate loss of vessel elasticity; or injury to muscle tissue, which generates a decrease in the contraction force of the muscles on the lymphatic vessels, impairing the muscle pump (EZZO *et al.*, 2016; ABBASI *et al.*, 2018).

Gritsenko *et al.* (2015) stated that 62% of women within one year of diagnosis developed lymphoedema, and 77% of women after three years, the condition persisted high up to ten years after surgery, indicating the need for persistent vigilance in lymphoedema care.

According to Sehl *et al.* (2013) after the end of cancer treatment, women experience a decrease in quality of life and an increase in functional limitations, factors that are aggravated in women over 65.

In the author's study, Mendes *et al.* (2014) carried out a descriptive-exploratory study with a quantitative approach, with the aim of characterizing the influence of the pain syndrome after mastectomy, correlating pain and quality of life.

The authors stated that the emotional aspect directly influences quality of life, and factors such as anxiety, cognitive fatigue, sleep disorders and depression may be correlated (MENDES et al., 2014).

2.1 PHYSIOTHERAPY ASSESSMENT

This topic highlights the importance of physiotherapy in the treatment of clinical complications following breast cancer, prevention and diagnosis of lymphoedema, using critical assessment criteria and specific therapeutic resources.

Figure 2 summarizes a sequence for physiotherapeutic assessment based on clinical evidence.

Figure 2: Outline of physiotherapy assessment after breast cancer.

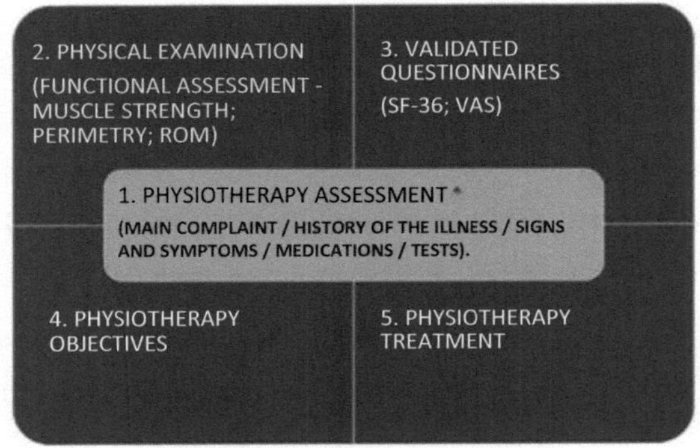

Source: author.

The physiotherapy assessment begins with obtaining personal data and a detailed anamnesis, including the main complaint and the history of the disease. It is important to ask about the type of surgery (quadrantectomy, tumorectomy or mastectomy), the date on which medical treatment began, the side operated on, axillary lymph node removal and which levels (axillary lymphadenectomy), hormone therapy, chemotherapy and/or radiotherapy.

In the post-operative evaluation, scar analysis is carried out by inspecting color, texture, temperature, presence of adherence, edema, keloid, pain, local hyperemia, among other factors.

With regard to the presence of lymphedema, the patient is initially asked about the sensation of heaviness in the upper limbs and clothing marks on the limb. The therapist will then carry out a thorough assessment of clinical signs such as changes in color, time of evolution of the edema, edema with a locker (Goted's sign), edema without a locker (Stemmer's sign), changes in sensitivity and temperature, as well as measuring the perimetry of the upper limbs.

The applicability of scales and clinical questionnaires, both of which are said to be subjective, are supported in the literature as resources that are easy to use, low cost and clinically relevant. However, the literature emphasizes the use of biomechanical and neurophysiological methods with quantitative data, which together complement the understanding of the clinical condition and the effects of treatments (ZHANG *et al.*, 2012; BUNEVICIUS, 2017).

The experience of pain is multidimensional, dynamic and involves psychological, cognitive, physiological and behavioral determinants, and the patient's self-report of pain intensity is the primary basis for assessment (BANOZIC *et al.,* 2018).

Numerous tools have been validated in the current literature with the aim of verifying the presence of pain, quantifying the severity and the level of reliability of the scales, including visual analog scales, numerical rating scales, verbal scales, symbols, among others. However, the appropriate selection of the scale must take into account the individual's cognitive state, level of consciousness, education and culture (AMERICAN PAIN SOCIETY, 2016).

According to the American Pain Society's Guideline for the Management of Postoperative Pain (2016), it is recommended that healthcare professionals apply pain assessment scales to track therapeutic responses and adjust treatment plans, as a reference to the progress or deterioration of pain management and its impact.

The SF-36 questionnaire (*Medical Outcomes Study 36 - Item Short-Form Health Survey*) is commonly used in health research to document the impact of the general health of individuals with different diagnoses, the severity of the disease or the effectiveness of interventions over time. Considered a valid and concise generic instrument, the SF-36 questionnaire provides a quantitative picture of an individual's state of health, determining their quality of life (TEHRANI *et al.*, 2011; ZHANG *et al.,* 2012).

Studies have shown a complex correlation between the frequent physical and psychological symptoms following breast cancer, such as anxiety, cognitive fatigue, sleep disorders and depression, which negatively interfere with quality of life and contribute to increased morbidity and mortality. In this sense, assessing the quality of life of women after breast cancer becomes fundamental in the management of patient care (MORO-VALDEZATE *et al.*, 2013; LANZA *et al.,* 2015).

Bunevicius (2017) states that the SF-36 questionnaire is considered the most widely used generic assessment tool in the world, applied mainly to cancer patients.

In another study by the author, Mendes *et al.* (2017) carried out a descriptive cross-sectional study with an exploratory nature with 105 post-breast cancer women, with the aim of comparing the quality of life using the SF-36 between women who had undergone mastectomy and conservative surgery to remove breast cancer.

Goniometry is considered the gold standard for assessing motor function. It is an easy-to-use, non-invasive and low-cost technique used to measure joint range of motion (TAJALI *et al.*, 2016).

Koehler *et al.* (2015) carried out a prospective cohort study with patients after breast cancer, in which they assessed shoulder abduction range of motion using goniometry, pain using the visual analog scale, and post-operative edema using perimetry to obtain limb circumference values.

Melchiorri *et al.* (2017) carried out a retrospective observational study with 64 women after unilateral mastectomy, and assessed late arm failure using a functional assessment scale, the SF-36 quality of life questionnaire and muscle strength using a manual strength dynamometer.

The assessment of motor function is important to quantify the degree of motor dysfunction, as well as the clinical outcome of the intervention used, in order to provide the physiotherapist with guidance on establishing the therapeutic approach. The use of biomedical instruments in clinical assessment, for example electromyography and dynamometry, are considered a prerequisite for the development of effective approaches (LI *et al.*, 2017).

2. 2 PHYSIOTHERAPY TREATMENT

Evidence has shown that rehabilitation has become an integral part of clinical care after breast cancer, through exercises that contribute to motor improvement and quality of life during the period of cancer treatment, as well as recovery after treatment (MORONE *et al.*, 2014; GOKAL *et al.*, 2015). Stout *et al.* (2012) reported the importance of early physiotherapeutic intervention, before the onset of functional limitations.

Physiotherapy started early focuses on preventing complications such as lymphoedema, retractions and shoulder dysfunction, as well as encouraging the patient to resume their daily activities, with physiotherapeutic interventions at all stages of cancer treatment through appropriate clinical assessment (GROEF *et al.*, 2015; OLIVEIRA *et al.*, 2016).

Initially, patients are instructed on skin care, which should be used routinely, through guidance and education on moisturizing the skin, preventing injuries, cuts and mycoses, excessive heat, needles and restrictive clothing on the affected limb (MCKEY; ALAPPATTU, 2015).

Deep massage techniques such as rubbing, sliding and S-shaped maneuvers are indicated because they promote tissue mobilization in conditions where tissue contracture and adherence cause pain and restriction of range of motion, such as axillary or lymphatic cord syndrome (LEWIS; CUNNINGHAM, 2016).

Sensitivity and scarring changes, due to skin retraction caused by the surgical procedure, are addressed by desensitization with different textures and temperatures, mobilization, stretching, flexibility, manual therapy and local massage to release the retracted tissue (WILSON, 2017).

Therapeutic exercises that encompass the muscle chain of the shoulder girdle provide positive effects, such as improved muscle mass, metabolic demand, microcirculation of the systems, skeletal muscle pumping, venous lymphatic reflux mechanism, flexibility and muscle strength, contributing to stabilization, joint mobility, and consequently improved range of motion (PARK, 2016).

According to Alpozgen *et al.* (2016), the shoulder exercise program consists of stretching and strengthening involving active and assisted active movements of flexion, extension, abduction, internal and external rotation of the shoulder joint, followed by isotonic resistance exercises with weights and elastic bands.

Corroborating the study, Groef *et al.* (2015) stated that assisted active mobilization exercises, active, stretching, scapulothoracic exercises and strengthening exercises to restore strength are necessary and should be started in the immediate postoperative period to encourage the performance of activities of daily living.

Complex Decongestive Therapy (CDT) is considered the gold standard in lymphedema management care. CDT is divided into two phases and includes the techniques of manual lymphatic drainage, multilayer compression, skin care, combined therapeutic exercises and patient training for self-application (EZZO *et al.,* 2016; HANSDORFER-KORZON *et al.,* 2016).

Phase I aims to reduce swelling through manual lymphatic drainage and compression with bandages, followed by advice on how to keep the skin healthy and free from infection, as well as a series of therapeutic exercises. Compression therapy is carried out using multi-layered bandages on the affected limb, consisting of gauze to wrap the fingers and hands, a stockinette sleeve to protect the skin and two or three layers of high-density foam (EZZO *et al.*, 2016).

Phase II is instituted after the volume of the limb has been reduced, with the aim of maintaining it through compression. The patient is instructed to wear sleeves with or without hand gloves, followed by home guidance on exercises, skin care and self-administered lymphatic drainage (EZZO *et al.*, 2016).

However, some authors emphasize that the available literature on DCT is still scarce, and the results of randomized controlled trials are limited and contradictory (BURAGADDA *et al.*, 2015; HAN *et al.,* 2016).

Tambour *et al.* (2014) stated that scientific evidence on the types of treatments and their combinations is scarce in the literature, and that some factors influence such as guidance on home exercises, the patient's adherence to the technique and the lack of specialized professionals in the field.

On the subject of rehabilitation after breast cancer, Mendes et al. (2013) conducted a double-blind longitudinal clinical study to assess the effects of motor rehabilitation using virtual reality projection on pain intensity, scapular strength, myoelectric activity and shoulder joint range of women after breast cancer.

The authors concluded that the virtual reality projection software developed in the study promoted pain relief, increased shoulder joint range of motion, muscle fiber recruitment and, consequently, scapular strength in women after breast cancer (MENDES et al., 2013).

In the study by the author and collaborators, Mendes et al. (2016) evaluated the medium- and long-term effects of vibration therapy on pain intensity, range of motion and

movement, myoelectric activity and muscle strength of women with post-surgical breast cancer.

The results of the aforementioned study showed a trend towards a reduction in compensatory movements, which activated the muscle contraction mechanism, as well as an increase in scapular strength when compared to the control group, in addition to an attenuation of painful symptoms and an improvement in shoulder movements (MENDES et al., 2016).

Still on the author's line of research, in 2018 she defended her doctoral thesis in Biomedical Engineering on the new perspectives of the physiotherapeutic approach after breast cancer, encompassing the applicability of robotic rehabilitation and virtual reality therapy.

With this in mind, the author published a commentary in *Integrative Clinical Medicine* on technological innovation in oncology, explaining the importance of clinical research into new short- and long-term physiotherapeutic interventions after breast cancer. The author emphasized the rehabilitation of acute and chronic clinical complications according to the needs of each woman, including education, restoration of motor functions and preventive measures through new technologies that contribute to an adequate and complete clinical assessment, as well as innovations throughout the rehabilitation process (MENDES, 2018).

3. UROLOGICAL CANCER AND MEN'S HEALTH

The prostate is a gland of the male reproductive system, responsible for producing the seminal fluid that feeds the sperm, located below the bladder and anterior to the rectum, the size of a walnut, which surrounds part of the urethra (PEREZ et al., 2018).

Prostate cancer is the most common malignant neoplasm in men, accounting for 30% of all male cancers (PARK et al., 2018). In Brazil, 68,220 new cases of prostate cancer are estimated for the 2018/2019 biennium, with an estimated risk of 66.12 new cases per 100,000 men (MINISTÉRIO DA SAÙDE, 2018).

In the Southeast, the ten types of cancer estimated to be most prevalent in men are: prostate cancer (30,080 cases), colon and rectum (10,040 cases), trachea, bronchus and lung (8,290 cases), oral cavity (5.920 cases), stomach (5,800 cases), bladder (3,720 cases), esophagus (3,460 cases), larynx (2,620 cases), non-Hodgkin's lymphoma (2,610 cases) and leukemia (2,500 cases) (MINISTÉRIO DA SAÙDE, 2018).

The hallmarks of oncogenesis and the progression of prostate cancer are related to androgens and androgen receptor signaling. Current literature discusses the interactions between androgen receptors, angiogenesis, vascular endothelial growth factor and DNA modification (ANTONARAKIS, 2018).

Benign prostatic hyperplasia is characterized by the proliferation of prostatic cells, which can lead to chronic bladder obstruction, with consequent urinary retention, infections, hematuria, stones and renal failure (PETRILLO et al., 2018).

Benign prostatic hyperplasia affects approximately 50% of men between the ages of 60 and 70, and 50% of individuals diagnosed with hyperplasia have lower urinary tract symptoms, mainly weak flow and a feeling of incomplete emptying, as well as other complications (JUNG et al., 2018).

In advanced stages, the progression of the disease can cause invasion of adjacent structures, generating pain, urinary retention due to bladder and/or urethral invasion, obstruction of the rectum, rectourethral or retrovesical fistulas, and compression of the pelvic nerve (AL-ABDIN; AL-BEESHI, 2018).

According to D'Abronzo and Ghosh (2018) the development, growth and metastasis of prostate cancer is primarily correlated with androgen, in which androgen deprivation therapy is the first therapeutic option for metastatic prostate cancer.

Almeida and Pereira (2018) stated that androgen suppression therapy associated with primary treatment, such as radical prostatectomy or radiotherapy, is effective in controlling local progression of the disease.

Numerous treatment modalities for prostate cancer are currently available, including active surveillance, radical prostatectomy, radiotherapy, androgen deprivation therapy, brachytherapy or high-intensity ultrasound therapy. Among the surgical modalities, robotic-assisted surgery is innovative.

However, regardless of the approach, after surgery some side effects are eminent, such as voiding and sexual dysfunction (DEGHEILI; MANSOUR; NASR, 2018).

Treatment for prostate cancer is constantly evolving these days, however, excessive detection with consequent negligent treatment has made active surveillance necessary, a standard management strategy for individuals with low-risk cancer (DALL'ERA; DAVIES; EGGENER, 2018).

Active surveillance has been used more frequently for patients at low risk of prostate cancer to monitor the progression of the disease, due to the fact that most men at low risk do not progress to high risk, avoiding morbid invasive treatments.

Radical prostatectomy is the most common treatment used in patients with localized prostate cancer; however, other techniques are used, such as open radical prostatectomy, laparoscopic prostatectomy and robot-assisted prostatectomy. Regardless of the surgical technique, urinary incontinence and sexual dysfunction are significant, contributing to a worsening quality of life (Wang et al., 2014; PARK et al., 2018).

The risk factors for the development of urinary incontinence after prostatectomy can be related to age, body mass index, resection of the neurovascular bundle, anastomotic stenosis, prostatic volume, previous history of transurethral resection of the prostate, decreased membranous length of the urethra (CHUGHTAI et al., 2013).

These facts can be attributed to injury or impairment of the urethral sphincter and bladder dysfunction, for example, detrusor hyperactivity, feeling of incomplete filling and low bladder compliance (Wang et al., 2014).

Bhatt et al. (2018) compared transperineal prostate biopsy with transrectal ultrasound-guided prostate biopsy using validated questionnaires. The authors stated that pain was significantly higher after transrectal biopsy (86% vs 61%), and transperineal biopsy is better tolerated by patients, however, a higher incidence of urinary retention (16.7% vs 5.7%) and sexual dysfunction (p=0.001) was reported. The authors concluded that regardless of the type of biopsy, patients should be informed about the possible risks of each type due to the impact on quality of life.

PSA blood tests associated with clinical staging and the Gleason score are considered the standard for classifying the risk of developing prostate cancer as low, intermediate or high (CLOS-GARCIA et al., 2018).

Currently, screening protocols include rectal examination and analysis of serum PSA (Prostate Specific Antigen) levels. In cases of suspected tumor, the patient is referred for transrectal prostate biopsy, ultrasound and histopathological examination (AREF-ESHGHI et al., 2018).

PSA (Prostate-Specific Antigen) was described by Wang et al. (1979) and first applied by Stamey et al. (1987). The serum PSA level is a tumor marker used for screening, detection and monitoring of prostate cancer, which correlates with potential malignancy and tumor burden (YAMADA et al., 2018).

PSA is a serine protease produced and released by prostate epithelial cells, which is secreted as an inactive proenzyme (proPSA) in the seminal fluid and activated by multiple enzymes produced by the prostate, considered a significant predictor of prostate cancer. Serum PSA has several different molecular forms, such as free PSA, complexed PSA and total PSA (GLASS; DALLERA 2018).

It is currently the biomarker used in conjunction with the touch test to diagnose prostate cancer. Serum levels are considered elevated above 4.0 ng/mL, which correlates with prostate cancer and benign conditions such as prostatitis and benign prostatic hyperplasia (LIMA et al., 2017).

According to Louro et al. (2007) it is important to evaluate the density, speed, age-adjusted values and transition zone for PSA analysis in order to increase the specificity of the diagnosis.

Radiotherapy promotes anti-tumor immune reactions directed at the primary lesion and metastases, with an effect on the genetic expression of the tumor, potentiating cell apoptosis (ALMEIDA; PEREIRA, 2018).

Bedini et al. (2018) stated that patients with high inflammatory conditions are at high risk of severe fibrosis after radiotherapy in the pelvic region, which explains the variability of toxicity.

Goineau et al. (2018) stated that radiotherapy was well tolerated and quality of life maintained in the patients evaluated in the study. However, some symptoms were reported in a substantial proportion of patients, such as urinary and digestive toxicity, acute diarrhea, fatigue, decreased social, physical and cognitive functioning.

Functional clinical complications after prostate cancer include urinary incontinence, dysuria and altered urinary frequency. However, these complications are often poorly interpreted and defined, making it difficult to obtain the true incidence and impact on quality of life, which makes it necessary to inform the patient correctly and openly, in order to avoid subsequent regret (ALBKRI et al., 2018).

Patients with benign prostatic hyperplasia report nocturia, defined as the desire to urinate during the night, with reports of two or more urinations, which affects the quality of sleep, as they need to wake up 3 or 4 hours after falling asleep, affecting the deep sleep phase (MIOTLA et al., 2017).

Prostate cancer treatment can result in sexual impotence, urinary incontinence or both (AL-ABDIN; AL-BEESHI, 2018).

Lehto et al. (2018) stated that all therapeutic modalities of active prostate cancer treatment generate persistent negative effects on quality of life, in which 33-48% of patients reported symptoms up to 5 years later.

According to the authors, prostatectomy and radiotherapy caused urinary incontinence, and radiotherapy caused symptoms of urinary irritation and intestinal dysfunction. The patients interviewed reported that the treatment had a negative effect on their sex life (81-93%), sexual dysfunction (70-92%) and the end of sexual activity with their spouses (20% to 58%).

Sallami (2017) stated that definitive urinary continence occurs after 1 year of surgery, however, 10% of men do not achieve complete recovery. This condition of urinary incontinence is justified by the damage to anatomical structures, such as the striated sphincter at the apex of the prostate and the smooth sphincter located at the neck of the bladder, by mechanisms due to direct damage to the sphincter fibers, nerve damage or changes in the urethrovesical anastomosis.

Stress urinary incontinence in men is related to urethral sphincter dysfunction and/or changes in the axis of the urethra, usually caused after radical prostatectomy or transurethral resection of the prostate (TURP), neurological injuries or pelvic floor trauma (CHUNG; KATZ; LOVE, 2017).

The male urethral sphincter has two parts, composed of an inner layer of smooth muscle, which is located close to the bladder neck and an outer skeletal muscle layer, located distally on the membranous membrane. Thus, prostatectomy is said to damage both layers, causing urinary incontinence, detrusor overactivity and nerve damage (SATHIANATHEN et al., 2017).

The external urethral sphincter corresponds to the site of peak urethral closure pressure and surrounds the membranous urethra, responsible for ensuring continence after radical prostatectomy, in which it is possible to observe in the urethral pressure profilometry examination, a decrease in the maximum urethral closure pressure and functional length (PACIK; FEDORKO, 2017).

Prostatectomy results in damage to the arteries and cavernous nerves, causing sexual dysfunction and consequent loss of penile erection. Studies show that after surgery, erectile dysfunction affects 95% of men over 70, 50% between 55 and 65, and 15-29% under 55 (PEREZ et al., 2018).

Hamilton and Mirza (2014) reported an incidence of erectile dysfunction in up to 90% of men after prostate cancer surgery, and 20 to 80% after radiotherapy, which is considered the most common side effect.

Erectile dysfunction is defined as the inability to achieve or maintain an erection sufficient for satisfactory sexual performance for both partners (DOREY et al., 2004).

Erectile dysfunction is characterized by the failure of the vascular reflex mechanism, which cannot pump blood with sufficient pressure to the corpus cavernosum, and as a result the erection cannot be maintained. After prostatectomy, the muscle responsible for the rigidity phase of the erection, called the ischiocavernosus muscle, becomes weakened due to the use of the bladder catheter (PEREZ et al., 2018).

Injury to cavernous nerve fibers leads to a process of Wallerian degeneration, in which the normal connections of the nervous tissue to the corpus cavernosum are lost, suggesting an absence of neuroregulatory function in penile erection, and penile neuropathy may develop due to degeneration and atrophy of the cavernous tissue (BURNETT 2006).

According to Dorey et al. (2004) the muscles of the pelvic floor play an important role in sexual activity, as contractions of the ischiocavernosus and bulbocavernosus muscles increase intracavernous pressure, influencing penile rigidity, due to the bulbocavernosus muscle compressing the deep dorsal vein of the penis in order to prevent blood from flowing out of the engorged penis.

Treatment for erectile dysfunction includes the use of oral medications such as sildenafil, vardenafil and tadalafil; intracavernous injections with alprostadil, phentolamine or papaverine; and vacuum erection devices such as penile prostheses, semi-rigid and inflatable (HAMILTON; MIRZA, 2014).

3.1 PHYSIOTHERAPY ASSESSMENT

Urinary incontinence is characterized by the involuntary loss of urine. This complaint occurs in both sexes, but is more frequent in women. Although the pathophysiology is evident in both sexes, male incontinence is a condition resulting from prostate enlargement or due to lesions following surgery and/or radiotherapy.

Rehabilitation requires determining the type of urinary incontinence and the signs and symptoms involved in micturition control, as well as assessing the integrity of muscles, fasciae, motor control and behavioral factors.

In clinical practice, it is important to analyze laboratory tests, imaging tests such as ultrasound, urethrocystoscopy and magnetic resonance imaging, and a detailed urodynamic evaluation.

The urodynamics examination is a diagnostic method used for functional assessment of the middle and lower urinary tract. The findings of the urodynamics exam assess detrusor and sphincter function, using information obtained from flowmetry, cystometry and electromyography.

When inspecting the pelvic floor, it is important to note tenderness, bladder distension, obvious hernias or swelling and erythema, post-surgical scars, deformities, prolapses and hemorrhoids.

The muscle test should be carried out using a digital touch to analyze the tone of the external anal sphincter during voluntary anal contraction.

According to the interpretation of the muscle contraction, it is classified as decreased, increased or normal and the parameters of the Perfect Scale.

The therapist can then administer questionnaires relating to the impact on quality of life and advise the patient on the importance of filling in the voiding diary correctly.

In the author's practice, the voiding diary is used to obtain the following information: total volume, minimum volume, maximum volume, voiding frequency, losses and use of protection, in which the patient is instructed to fill in the diary at the beginning and every five sessions of physiotherapy treatment.

Manometry is used to quantify the muscle tone and contractility of the pelvic muscles using a pressure sensor. The test is carried out with a verbal command from the therapist asking for voluntary contraction and relaxation of the anal sphincter after positioning the probe (PEDRAZA et al., 2014).

The patient should be instructed to perform a series of voluntary contractions with consequent relaxation of the PFM, with repetitions and recordings at a specific time interval.

The aim of electromyography is to capture muscle activity. It can be performed with an internal rectal electrode and surface electrodes on accessory muscles, such as the rectus abdominis muscle, and a reference electrode for noise grounding positioned on the iliac bone.

Pedraza et al. (2014) described a protocol for collecting electromyography, highlighting the recordings in 4 phases: initial phase or baseline, in which the patient remains at rest for 60 seconds to determine baseline electromyographic activity, i.e. at rest; rapid contraction phase in which activity is recorded during five rapid physical contractions; contraction and tonic resistance, with electromyographic recording of the PFM and rectus abdominis, with sustained contraction and rest for 10 seconds each; and the late baseline phase, which assesses the patient at rest for 60 seconds.

The therapeutic resources, whether invasive or non-invasive, depend directly on the severity of the symptoms, and include: training of the pelvic floor muscles with the correct determination of the level of intensity, duration and frequency of the exercise, manometric or electromyographic biofeedback, electrostimulation, behavioral therapy and external penile compression devices.

3.2 PHYSIOTHERAPY TREATMENT

Interventions with myofascial release, stretching and exercises, biofeedback and neuromodulation are interventions that contribute positively to improving chronic pelvic pain syndrome and quality of life in men (MASTERSON et al., 2017).

According to the author's clinical practice, some techniques are essential in physiotherapy treatment, such as therapeutic exercises to improve pelvic mobility, flexibility and strengthening of the pelvic floor muscles, which can be associated with the use of biofeedback; pelvic electrostimulation or neuromodulation to reduce pain; and manual therapy techniques, such as manipulation of the pelvic floor and abdominal muscles; myofascial trigger point release.

The muscles of the pelvic floor are classified morphologically as skeletal muscles, which adapt to stress in the same way as the other muscles in this group. The external anal and urethral sphincter muscle and the bulbospongiosus muscle originate from the puborectalis muscle and act dependently on each other (RAJKOWSKA-LABON et al., 2014).

Good neuromuscular coordination has a positive influence on the normal function of the pelvic floor, due to the fact that the pelvic muscles have points of origin and insertion that are directly connected by bones, ligaments and fasciae.

However, some factors slow down muscle responses, such as advanced age, which is associated with slower response times due to the decreased ability of the urethra to contract against the pubic symphysis (RAJKOWSKA-LABON et al., 2014).

Resistance and strength training in patients with urinary incontinence aims to change muscle morphology, increasing diameter, improving neurological indices with a consequent increase in the number of active motor neurons and excitatory stimuli, contributing to improved muscle tone (RAJKOWSKA-LABON et al., 2014).

Pelvic floor muscle exercises help improve urinary control by increasing the strength, endurance and coordination of the pelvic muscles, as well as functionally activating the external sphincter of the urethra. Consequently, they generate hypertrophy of the periurethral striated muscles, with strengthening and stiffening of the pelvic floor muscles, connective tissues and the inhibitory reflex of the detrusor muscle (MINA et al., 2015).

The pelvic floor muscles are part of a lumbopelvic structural complex, which includes the muscles of the pelvic floor, respiratory diaphragm, transverse abdominis and lower spine, including the multifidus muscle (RAJKOWSKA-LABON et al., 2014).

Strategies for activating the pelvic floor muscles are based on isolated muscle tension, functional training, motor control, the use of muscle synergies involving the transverse abdominis muscle and correct breathing patterns.

Jung et al. (2016) compared the effects of abdominal contraction maneuvers, maximal expiration and maximal contraction of the pelvic muscles during bridge and abdominal exercises in healthy men and women. The authors affirm the importance of emphasizing maximal PFM contraction during trunk stabilization exercises, as they obtained better results during abdominal exercises when compared to bridge exercises.

Dorey et al. (2004) described a sequence of pelvic exercises for men with erectile dysfunction. The series included exercises in orthostatism, sedation, supine position, during walking, after urination, which were oriented towards sustained, maximal and submaximal contraction) and exercises during sexual activity and ejaculation.

Fernândez et al. (2014) carried out a meta-analysis to assess the evidence of pelvic muscle training on urinary incontinence after radical prostatectomy. The authors stated that performing three sets of 10 repetitions a day of PFM training contributes to improved continence after radical prostatectomy.

The use of biofeedback associated with pelvic floor exercises is used to promote improved continence after prostatectomy with good levels of scientific evidence (SANTOS et al., 2018).

Perez et al. (2018) stated that the use of biofeedback in the preoperative period of radical prostatectomy was effective in reducing urinary incontinence and erectile dysfunction.

In clinical practice, the association of biofeedback with pelvic muscle training has shown positive results, with an emphasis on increasing muscle strength and motivating the patient during therapy.

Biofeedback provides awareness of the isolated muscle activity of the pelvic floor in order to avoid co-contractions. Feedback on the correct contraction is signaled with sound or visual effects, in order to improve understanding and the ability to contract in subsequent activities.

Electrostimulation of the pelvic floor can be carried out using a probe connected to the equipment (TENS/FES), with the aim of promoting urethral closure by activating the PFM through stimulation of the pudendal nerve. It is believed that stimulation improves the denervated urethra and pelvic floor muscles, promoting the reinnervation process (CHUGHTAI et al., 2013).

In the application of electrostimulation, the author emphasizes the benefits of the technique in terms of increased motor recruitment and inhibition of detrusor hyperactivity, which can be applied in different combinations in each treatment session according to the patient's clinical condition and assessment.

Electrostimulation of the pudendal nerves produces maximum contraction of the pelvic floor, with consequent improvement in urethral closure and attenuation of detrusor hyperactivity.

Behavioral therapy includes prevention, control and self-monitoring strategies by means of a voiding diary, which is considered effective in the physiotherapeutic treatment of persistent urinary incontinence after prostatectomy (GOODE et al., 2011).

The author emphasizes the importance of behavioral therapy, mainly because it helps to reduce the frequency of urinary incontinence, urinary frequency, urgency and nocturia, advocating the association of the results with the patient's activities of daily living and quality of life.

Evidence shows that physical activity improves body composition, urinary incontinence, muscle strength, cardiorespiratory fitness, depression, fatigue and quality of life, with a consequent increase in survival in men with cancer (FOX et al., 2017).

Yunfeng et al. (2017) stated that physical exercise contributed significantly to improving muscle strength, exercise tolerance, body fat control, body mass index and sexual function in patients with prostate cancer.

4. THANKS

The author would like to thank the members of Clinica Spazio Saùde for all their support and admiration and the Universidade do Vale do Paraiba - Faculdade de Ciências da Saù - Ambulatòrio de Estàgio Supervisado em Uroginecologia.

5. REFERENCES

ABBASI, B., *et al*. The effect of relaxation techniques on edema, anxiety and depression in patients with post-mastectomy lymphedema undergoing comprehensive decongestant therapy: a clinical trial. **Plos One,** v. 13, n. 1, p. 2018.

ABELLO, A.; DAS, A. Electrical neuromodulation in the management of lower urinary tract dysfunction: evidence, experience and future prospects. **Ther. Adv. Urol.**, v. 10, n. 5, p. 165-173.

ADEMUYIWA, F. O.; ELLIS, M. J.; MA, C. X. Neoadjuvant therapy in operable breast cancer: application to triple negative breast cancer. **J. Oncol.**, v. 2013, p.1-8, 2013.

AL-ABDIN, O. Z.; AL-BEESHI, I. Z. Prostate cancer in the Arab population. **Saudi Med. J.**, v. 39, n. 5, p. 453- 458, 2018.

ALBKRI, A., et al. Urinary Incontinence, Patient Satisfaction, and Decisional Regret after Prostate Cancer Treatment: A French National Study. **Urol. Int.**, v. 100, p. 50-56, 2018.

ALMEIDA, P. L.; PEREIRA, B. J. Local Treatment of Metastatic Prostate Cancer: What is the Evidence So Far? **Hindawi Prostate Cancer**, v. 2018, p. 1-8, 2018.

ALPOZGEN, A. Z., *et al.* Effectiveness of Pilates-based exercises on upper extremity disorders related with breast cancer treatment. **Eur. J. Cancer Care**, v. 00, p. 1-8, 2016.

ALSAIF, A. Breast cancer recurrence after sentinel lymph node biopsy. **Pak J. Med. Sci.**, v. 31, n. 6, p. 1426-1431, 2015.

AL-SHAIKH, G., et al. Pessary use in stress urinary incontinence: a review of advantages, complications, patient satisfaction, and quality of life. **International Journal of Women's Health**, v. 10, p. 195-201, 2018.

AMERICAN PAIN SOCIETY. Guidelines on the Management of Postoperative Pain. **J. of Pain**, v. 17, n. 2, p. 131-157, 2016.

AMORIM, A. C., et al. Effect of combined actions of hip adduction/abduction on the force generation and maintenance of pelvic floor muscles in healthy women. **PLoS One**, v. 12, n. 5, p. 1-12, 2017.

ANDRADE, R. L., et al. An education program about pelvic floor muscles improved women's knowledge but not pelvic floor muscle function, urinary incontinence or sexual function: a randomized trial. **Journal of Physiotherapy**, v. 64, n. 2018, p. 91-96, 2018.

ANGELO, P. H., et al. A manometry classification to assess pelvic floor muscle function in women. **Plos One**, v. 12, n. 10, p. 1-8, 2017.

ANTONARAKIS, E. S. AR Signaling in Human Malignancies: Prostate Cancer and Beyond. **Cancers**, v. 10, n. 22, p. 1-3, 2018.

AOKI, Y., et al. Urinary incontinence in women. **Nat Rev Dis Primers**, v. 3, n. 17042, p. 1-41, 2018.

AREF-ESHGHI, E., et al. Genomic DNA Methylation-Derived Algorithm Enables Accurate Detection of Malignant Prostate. **Front. Oncol.**, v. 8, n. 100, 2018.

BAKKER, R. M., et al. Sexual Rehabilitation After Pelvic Radiotherapy and Vaginal Dilator Use - Consensus Using the Delphi Method. **Int J Gynecol Cancer,** v. 24, n. 8, p. 14991506, 2014.

BANOZIC, A., *et al.* Neuroticism and pain catastrophizing aggravate response to pain in healthy adults: an experimental study. **J. Pain,** v. 31, n. 1, p. 16-26, 2018.

BEDINI, N., et al. Evaluation of Mediators Associated with the Inflammatory Response in Prostate Cancer Patients Undergoing Radiotherapy. **Hindawi Disease Markers**, v. 2018, n. 1-9, 2018.

BEN-AHARON, I., et al. Premature ovarian aging in BRCA carriers: a prototype of systemic precocious aging? **Oncotarget,** v. 9, n. 22, p. 15931-15941, 2018.

BEYAZ, S. G., *et al.* Postmastectomy pain: a cross-sectional study of prevalence, pain characteristics, and effects on quality of life. **Chin. Med. J.**, v. 129, n. 1, p. 66-71, 2016.

BHATT, N. R., et al. Patient experience after transperineal template prostate biopsy compared to prior transrectal ultrasound guided prostate biopsy. **Cent. European J. Urol.**, v. 71, p. 43-47, 2018.

BHATTA, S., *et al.* Factors associated with compliance to adjuvant hormone therapy in black and white women with breast cancer. **SpringerPlus**, v. 2, n. 356, p. 1-7, 2013.

BHATTARAI, A; STAAT, M. Modelling of Soft Connective Tissues to Investigate Female

Pelvic Floor Dysfunctions. **Computational and Mathematical Methods in Medicine**, v. 2018, p. 1-16, 2017.

BOGANI, G.; DITTO, A.; MARTINELLI, F.; SIGNORELLI, M.; PEROTTO, S.; LORUSSO, D.; RASPAGLIESI, F. A critical assessment on the role of sentinel node mapping in endometrial cancer. **Journal Gynecologic Oncology**, v. 26, n. 4, p. 252-254, 2015.

BRACKSTONE, M. A review of the literature and discussion: establishing a consensus for the definition of post-mastectomy pain syndrome to provide a standardized clinical and research approach. **J. Can. Chir.**, v. 59, n. 5, p. 294-295, 2016.

BRENNER, D. R., *et al.* Breast cancer survival among young women: a review of the role of modifiable lifestyle factors. **Cancer Causes Control,** v. 27, p. 459-472, 2016.

BUNEVICIUS, A. Reliability and validity of the SF-36 Health Survey Questionnaire in patients with brain tumors: a cross-sectional study. **Health Qual. Life Outcomes,** v. 15, n. 9, p. 1-7, 2017.

BURAGADDA, S., *et al.* Effect of complete decongestive therapy and a home program for patients with post mastectomy lymphedema. **J. Phys. Ther. Sci., v.** 27, p. 2743-2748, 2015.

CARTER, J.; HUANG, H; CHASE, D. M.; WALKER, J. L; CELLA, D.; WENZEL, L. Sexual Function of Endometrial Cancer Patients Enrolled on the Gynecologic Oncology Group LAP2 Study. **International Journal of Gynecological Cancer**, v. 22, v. 9, p. 1624-1633, 2012.

CHEN, J. Q.; WU, Z.; WEN, L.; MIAO, J. Z.; HU, Y.; XUE, R. Preoperative and postoperative analgesic techniques in the treatment of patients undergoing transabdominal hysterectomy: a preliminary randomized trial. **BMC Anesthesiology**, v. 15, n. 70, p. 1-7, 2015.

CHEN, M. N., et al. The bidirectional association among female hormone-related cancers: breast, ovary, and uterine corpus. **Cancer Medicine**, 2018.

CHENG, H., *et al.* A systematic review and meta-analysis of harmonic technology compared with conventional techniques in mastectomy and breast-conserving surgery with lymphadenectomy for breast cancer. **Dove Med. Press Breast Cancer**, v. 8, p. 125140, 2016.

CHEVALIER, F.; FERNANDEZ-LAO, C; CUESTA-VARGAS, A. I. Normal reference values of strength in pelvic floor muscle of women: a descriptive and inferential study. **BMC Women's Health**, v. 14, n. 143, p. 1-9, 2014.

CHOI, K. H., et al. Clinical impact of boost irradiation to pelvic lymph node in uterine cervical cancer treated with definitive chemoradiotherapy. **Medicine,** v. 97, n. 16, p. 19, 2018.

CHUGHTAI, B., et al. Conservative Treatment for Postprostatectomy Incontinence. **Rev Urol.**, v. 15, n. 2, p.61-66, 2013.

CHUNG, E.; KATZ, D. J.; LOVE, C. Adult male stress and urge urinary incontinence - A review of pathophysiology and treatment strategies for voiding dysfunction in men. **Reprinted From Afp**, v. 46, n. 9, p. 661-666, 2017.

CLAYTON, A. H., et al. Evaluation and Management of Hypoactive Sexual Desire Disorder. **Sex Med.**, v. 6, n. 59, p. 59-74, 2018.

CLOS-GARCIA, M., et al. Metabolic alterations in urine extracellular vesicles are associated with prostate cancer pathogenesis and progression. Journal of Extracellular Vesicles, v. 7, p. 1-15, 2018.

COOK, M. S., et al. Age-related alterations in female obturator internus muscle. **Int. Urogynecol. J.**, v. 28, n. 5, p. 729-734, 2017.

D'ABRONZO, L. S.; GHOSH, P. M. eIF4E Phosphorylation in Prostate Cancer. **Neoplasia**, v. 20, n. xx, p. 563-573, 2018.

DALL'ERA, M. A.; DAVIES, B.; EGGENER, S. Active surveillance for prostate cancer. **Transl. Androl. Urol.**, v. 7, n. 2, p. 195-196, 2018.

DEGHEILI, J. A.; MANSOUR, M. M.; NASR, R. W. Symphysis Pubis Osteomyelitis: An Uncommon Complication after Robotic Assisted Radical Prostatectomy-Case

Description with Literature Review. **Hindawi Case Reports in Urology**, v. 2018, p. 1-5, 2018.

DOREY, G., et al. Randomized controlled trial of pelvic floor muscle exercises and manometric biofeedback for erectile dysfunction. **British Journal of General Practice**, v. 54, p. 819-825, 2014.

EZZO, J., *et al.* Manual lymphatic drainage for lymphedema following breast cancer treatment. **Cochrane Database Syst. Rev.**, v. 5, p. 1-73, 2016.

FERNANDEZ, R. A., et al. Improvement of Continence Rate with Pelvic Floor Muscle Training PostProstatectomy: A Meta-Analysis of Randomized Controlled Trials. **Urol. Int.**, v. 94, p. 125-132, 2015.

FOX, L., et al. Real World Evidence: A Quantitative and Qualitative Glance at Participant Feedback from a Free-Response Survey Investigating Experiences of a Structured Exercise Intervention for Men with Prostate Cancer. **Hindawi BioMed Research International**, v. 2017, p. 1-10, 2017.

FUJISAKI, A., et al. Influence of adequate pelvic floor muscle contraction on the movement of the coccyx during pelvic floor muscle training. **J. Phys. Ther. Sci.**, v. 30, p. 544-548, 2018.

GILBERT, E.; USSHER, J. M.; PERTZ, J. Sexuality after gynaecological cancer: A review of the material, intrapsychic, and discursive aspects of treatment on women's sexual- wellbeing. **Maturitas**, v. 70, n. 2011, p. 42- 57, 2011.

GLASS, A. S.; DALL'ERA, M. A. Indications for and transitioning to secondary treatment while on active surveillance for prostate cancer. **Transl. Androl. Urol.**, v. 7, n. 2, p. 236242, 2018.

GOODE, P. C., et al. Behavioral Therapy With or Without Biofeedback and Pelvic Floor Electrical

Stimulation for Persistent Post-Prostatectomy Incontinence - A Randomized Controlled Trial. **JAMA**, v. 12, n. 305, p. 151-159, 2011.

GOINEAU, A., et al. Comprehensive Geriatric Assessment and quality of life after localized prostate cancer radiotherapy in elderly patients. **Plos One**, v. 13, n. 4, p. 1-14, 2018.

GOKAL, K., *et al.* Can physical activity help to maintain cognitive functioning and psychosocial well-being among breast cancer patients treated with chemotherapy? A randomized controlled trial: study protocol. **B. M. C. Public Health**, v. 15, n. 414, p. 1-8, 2015.

GOKTAS, S. B.; GUN, I.; YILDIZ, M. N.; SAKAR, M. N.; CAGLAYAN, S. The effect of total hysterectomy on sexual function and depression. **Pakistan Journal of Medical Sciences**, v. 31, n. 3, p. 700-705, 2015.

GRITSENKO, V., *et al.* Feasibility of using low-cost motion capture for automated screening of shoulder motion limitation after breast cancer surgery. **Plos One**, v. 10, n. 6, p. 1-9, 2015.

GROEF, A., *et al.* Effectiveness of postoperative physical therapy for upper limb impairments following breast cancer treatment: a systematic review. **Arch. Phys. Med. Rehabil.**, v. 96, n. 6, p. 1140-1153, 2015.

GROVER, S.; HILL-KAYSER, C. E.; VACHANI, C.; HAMPSHIRE, M. K.; DILULLO, G. A.; METZ, J. A. Patient reported late effects of gynecological cancer treatment. **Gynecologic Oncology**, v. 124, n. 2012, p. 399-403, 2012.

GUNER, O., et al. An examination of the sexual functions of patients who underwent a gynecologic cancer operation and received brachytherapy. **Pak J. Med. Sci.**, v. 34, n. 1, p. 15-19, 2018.

HAMILTON, Z.; MIRZA, M. Post-prostatectomy erectile dysfunction: contemporary approaches from a US perspective. **Research and Reports in Urology**, v. 6, p. 35-41, 2014.

HAN, C., *et al.* The Feasibility and Oncological Safety of Axillary Reverse Mapping in Patients with Breast Cancer: A Systematic Review and Meta-Analysis of Prospective Studies. **Plos One**, v. 11, n. 2, p. 1-16, 2016.

HAN, C.; YANG, L.; ZUO, W. A mini-review on factors and countermeasures associated with false-negative sentinel lymph node biopsies in breast cancer. **Chin. J. Cancer Res.**, v. 28, n. 3, p. 370-376, 2016.

HANSDORFER-KORZON, R., *et al.* Are compression corsets beneficial for the treatment of breast cancer-related lymphedema? New opportunities in physiotherapy treatment - a preliminary report. **Onco. Targets Ther.**, v. 2016, n. 9, p. 2089-2098, 2016.

HENTZE, J. L., et al. Searching for new biomarkers in ovarian cancer patients: Rationale and design of a retrospective study under the Mermaid III Project. **Contemporary Clinical Trials Communications**, v. 8, n. 2017, p. 167-174, 2017.

HEYDARI, F.; MOTAGHED, Z.; ABBASZADEH, S. Relationship between hysterectomy and severity of female stress urinary incontinence. **Electronic Physician**, v. 9, n. 6, p. 46784682, 2017.

HILL, A.; ALAPPATTU, M. Quality-of-Life Outcomes Following Surface Electromyography Biofeedback as an Adjunct to Pelvic Floor Muscle Training for Urinary Incontinence: A Case Report. **J Womens Health Phys Therap**, v. 41, n. 2, p. 73-82, 2018.

HWANG, E. S., *et al.* Survival after lumpectomy and mastectomy for early stage invasive breast cancer: the effect of age and hormone receptor status. **Cancer**, v. 119, n. 7, p. 1402-1411, 2013.

JERZAK, K., *et al.* Does adjuvant radiation therapy benefit women with small mammography-detected breast cancers? **Curr. Oncol.**, v. 24, n. 1, p. 28-32, 2017.

JUNG, H., et al. Comparison of changes in the mobility of the pelvic floor muscle on during the abdominal drawing-in maneuver, maximal expiration, and pelvic floor muscle maximal contraction. **J. Phys. Ther. Sci.**, v. 28, p. 467-472, 2016.

JUNG, J. H., et al. The association of benign prostatic hyperplasia with lower urinary tract stones in adult men: A retrospective multicenter study. **Asian Journal of Urology,** v. 5, p. 118-121, 2018.

KANAO, H.; FUJIWARA, K.; EBISAWA, K.; HADA, T.; OTA, Y.; ANDOU, M. Various types of total laparoscopic nerve-sparing radical hysterectomies and their effects on bladder function**. Journal of Gynecologic Oncology**, v. 25, n. 3, p. 198-205, 2014.

KARKHANIS, P.; PATEL, A.; GALAAL, K. Urinary tract fistulas in radical surgery for cervical cancer: The importance of early diagnosis. **EJSO The Journal of Cancer Surgery**, v. 38, p. 943-947, 2012.

KASHANIAN, M., et al. Evaluation of the effect of pelvic floor muscle training (PFMT or Kegel exercise) and assisted pelvic floor muscle training (APFMT) by a resistance device (Kegelmaster device) on urinary incontinence in women: a randomized trial. **European Journal of Obstetrics & Gynecology and Reproductive Biology**, v. 159, n. 2011, p. 218223, 2011.

KATO, K.; TATE, S.; NISHIKIMI, K.; SHOZU, M. Bladder function after modified posterior exenteration for primary gynecological cancer. **Gynecologic Oncology**, v. 129, n. 2013, p. 229-233, 2013.

KHOSHBATEN, μ., et al. Irritable bowel syndrome in women undergoing hysterectomy and tubular ligation. **Gastroenterology and Hepatology From Bed to Bench**, v. 4, n. 3, p. 138-141, 2011.

KIM, H. S., et al. Conventional versus nerve-sparing radical surgery for cervical cancer: a meta-analysis. **Journal of Gynecological Oncology**, v. 26, n. 2, p. 100-110, 2015.

KIM, S. W., et al. Management of a patient with vesicocutaneous fistula presenting 13 years after radiotherapy performed for cervical cancer. **Turk J. Urol**., v. 44, n. 2, p. 1858, 2018.

KOEHLER, L. A., *et al.* Movement, Function, Pain, and Postoperative Edema in Axillary Web Syndrome. **Phys. Ther.**, v. 95, n. 10, p. 1345-1353, 2015.

KOMISARUK, B. R.; FRANGOS, E.; WHIPPLE, B. Hysterectomy improves sexual response? Addressing a crucial omission in the literature. **Journal of Minimally Invasive Gynecology**, v. 18, n. 3, p. 288-295, 2011.

KUPERMAN, N. S.; RUSSOMANO, F. B.; MELO, Y. L. M. F.; GOMES, S. C. S. Preinvasive and invasive disease in women with cytological diagnosis of high-grade lesion and high-grade lesion cannot exclude microinvasion. **BMC Women's Health**, v. 15, n. 81, p. 1-6, 2015.

LANZA, M., *et al.* Quality of life and volume reduction in women with secondary lymphoedema related to breast cancer. **Int. J. Cancer**, v. 2015, p. 1-6, 2015.

LARSSON, I. M.; SORENSEN, J. A.; BILLE, C. The Post-mastectomy Pain Syndrome-A Systematic Review of the Treatment Modalities. Breast J., v. XX, n. XX, p. 1-6, 2017.

LAU, H. H.; HUANG, W. C.; SU, T. H. Urinary leakage during sexual intercourse among women with incontinence: Incidence and risk factors. **Plos One**, v. 12, n. 5, p. 1-8, 2017.

LEE, W. Patients' perception and adherence to vaginal dilator therapy: a systematic review and synthesis employing symbolic interactionism. **Patient Preference and Adherence**, v. 2018, n. 12, p. 551-560, 2018.

LEHTO, U. S., et al. Patients' perceptions of the negative effects following different prostate cancer treatments and the impact on psychological well-being: a nationwide survey. British Journal of Cancer, v. 116, p. 864-873, 2017.

LESURF, R., *et al.* Molecular features of subtype-specific progression from ductal carcinoma in situ to invasive breast cancer. **Cell Reports**, v. 16, p.1-14, 2016.

LEVIN, A. O., et al. Sexual Morbidity Associated With Poorer Psychological Adjustment Among. **Gynecological Cancer Survivors**, v. 20, n. 3, 1-18, 2010.

LEWIS, P. A.; CUNNINGHAM, J. E. Dynamic Angular Petrissage as Treatment for Axillary Web Syndrome Occurring after Surgery for Breast Cancer: a Case Report. **Int. J. Ther. Massage Bodywork,** v. 9, n. 2, p. 28-37, 2016.

LI, F., et al. Urological complications after radical hysterectomy with postoperative radiotherapy and radiotherapy alone for cervical cancer. **Medicine**, v. 97, n. 13, p. 1-5, 2018.

LI, Y., *et al.* Herbal Medicine for Hot Flushes Induced by Endocrine Therapy in Women with Breast Cancer: A Systematic Review and Meta-Analysis. **J. Evid. Based Complementary Altern. Med.,** v. 2016, p. 1-11, 2016.

LI, Y., *et al.* Motor function evaluation of hemiplegic upper-extremities using data fusion from wearable inertial and surface EMG sensors. **Sensors,** v. 17, n. 582, p. 1-17, 2017.

LIMA, A. R., et al. Discrimination between the human prostate normal and cancer cell exometabolome by GC-MS. **Scientific Reports**, v. 8, p. 5539, 2017.

LIMA, R. V., et al. Female Sexual Function in Women with Suspected Deep Infiltrating Endometriosis. Rev. Bras. Ginecol. Obstet., v. 40, p. 115-120, 2018.

LOBBEZOO, D., *et al.* The role of histological subtype in hormone receptor positive metastatic breast cancer: similar survival but different therapeutic approaches. **Oncotarget**, v. 7, n. 20, p. 29412-29419, 2016.

LOPES, T. C. R., *et al.* Mammographic screening of women attending a reference service center in southern Brazil. **Asian Pac. J. Cancer Prev.**, v. 17, n. 3, p. 1385-1391, 2016.

LOURO, N., et al. Comparative evaluation of total PSA, free PSA/total PSA and complexed PSA in the detection of prostate cancer. **Acta Urològica**, v. 24, n. 1, p. 3944, 2007.

LUCENTE, V., et al. Biomechanical paradigm and interpretation of female pelvic floor conditions before a treatment. **International Journal of Women's Health**, v. 2017, n. 9, p. 521-550, 2017.

LUPIA, M.; CAVALLARO, U. Ovarian cancer stem cells: still an elusive entity? **Molecular Cancer**, v. 16, n. 64, p. 1-17, 2017.

MACON, M. B.; FENTON, S. E. Endocrine disruptors and the breast: early life effects and later life disease. **J. Mammary Gland. Biol.**, v. 18, n. 1, p. 1-33, 2013.

MAESHIMA, Y., *et al.* Experience with Bilateral Risk-Reducing Mastectomy for an Unaffected BRCA Mutation Carrier. **J. Breast Cancer,** n. 19, v. 2, p. 218-221, 2016.

MANCHANA, T. Long-term Lower Urinary Tract Dysfunction in Gynecologic Cancer Survivors. **Asian**

Pacific Journal of Cancer Prevention, v. 12, p. 285-288, 2011.

MARGAN, M. M., *et al.* Molecular portrait of the normal human breast tissue and its influence on breast carcinogenesis. **J. Breast Cancer,** n. 19, v. 2, p. 99-111, 2016.

MARIN, F., et al. Postoperative surgical complications of lymphadenohysterocolpectomy. **Journal of Medicine Life**, v. 7, n. 1, p. 60-66, 2014.

MARQUES, A. A.; SILVA, P. P.; AMARAL, M. T. P. **Treatise on Physiotherapy in Women's Health.** Roca, 2011.

MARTINHO, N. M., et al. Intra and inter-rater reliability study of pelvic floor muscle dynamometric measurements. **Braz. J. Phys. Ther.**, v. 19, n. 2, p. 97-104, 2015.

MASTERSON, T. A., et al. Comprehensive pelvic floor physical therapy program for men with idiopathic chronic pelvic pain syndrome: a prospective study. **Transl Androl Urol.**, v. 6, n. 5, p. 910-915, 2017.

MAXWELL, M., et al. PROPEL: implementation of an evidence based pelvic floor muscle training intervention for women with pelvic organ prolapse: a realist evaluation and outcomes study protocol. **BMC Health Services Research**, v. 17, n. 843, p. 1-10, 2017.

MCKEY, K. P.; ALAPPATTU, M. J. Physical Therapy Intervention to Augment Outcomes Of Lymph Node Transfer Surgery for a Breast Cancer Survivor with Secondary Upper Extremity Lymphedema: A Case Report. **Int. J. Stud. Scholarsh Phys. Ther.**, v. 1, n. 3044, p. 1-27, 2015.

MELCHIORRI, G., *et al.* New approach to evaluate late arm impairment and effects of dragon boat activity in breast cancer survivors. **Medicine,** v. 96, n. 44, p. 1-8, 2017.

MENDES, I. S. Study of the clinical applicability of vibration blankets and virtual reality in secondary complications of breast cancer. **Master's dissertation.** University of Vale do Paraiba, 2013.

MENDES, I. S., *et al.* Correlation of pain and quality of life in women after breast cancer surgery. **Mundo Saùde**, v. 38, n. 2, p. 189-196, 2014.

MENDES, I. S., et al. Effects of vibration therapy in the musculoskeletal system in post-surgical breast cancer women: longitudinal controlled clinical study. **Res. Biomed. Eng.**, v. 32, n. 3, p. 213-222, 2016.

MENDES, I. S., *et al.* Impact of mastectomy and breast-conserving surgery on quality of life of women after breast cancer. **O Mundo da Saùde,** v. 41, n. 4, p. 703-710, 2017.

MENDES, I. L. Innovation Oncological Rehabilitation: Applicability of the Different Techniques

Physiotherapeutic Post Breast Cancer. **Int. Clin. Med.**, v. 2, n. 1, p. 1-2, 2018.

MINA, D. S., et al. A pilot randomized trial of conventional versus advanced pelvic floor exercises to treat urinary incontinence after radical prostatectomy: a study protocol. **BMC Urology**, v. 15, n. 94, p. 1-10, 2015.

MINISTRY OF HEALTH. José Alencar Gomes da Silva National Cancer Institute (INCA). **Estimate 2016 - Incidence of Cancer in Brazil**. Rio de Janeiro: INCA; 2015.

MINISTRY OF HEALTH. José Alencar Gomes da Silva National Cancer Institute (INCA).

Estimate 2018 - Cancer Incidence in Brazil. Rio de Janeiro: INCA; 2018.

MIOTLA, P., et al. Diagnostic and therapeutic recommendations for patients with nocturia. **Cent European J Urol**, v. 70, p. 388-393, 2017.

MOHKTAR, M. S., et al. A quantitative approach to measure women's sexual function using electromyography: A preliminary study of the Kegel exercise. **Med Sci Monit.**, v. 19, p. 1159-1166, 2013.

MORONE, G., *et al*. Effects of a multidisciplinary educational rehabilitative intervention in breast cancer survivors: the role of body image on quality of life outcomes. **Sci. World J. Journal**, v. 2014, p. 1-11, 2014.

MORO-VALDEZATE, D., *et al*. Evolution of health-related quality of life in breast cancer patients during the first year of follow-up. **J. Breast Cancer,** n. 16, n. 1, p. 104-111, 2013.

MOSLEHI, R., *et al*. Importance of hereditary and selected environmental risk factors in- the etiology of inflammatory breast cancer: a case-comparison study. **B. M. C. Cancer,** v. 16, n. 334, p. 1-9, 2016.

MOTA, R. L. Female urinary incontinence and sexuality. **Int. Braz. J. Urol.**, v. 43, p. 2028, 2017.

NORONHA, A. F., et al. Treatments for invasive carcinoma of the cervix: what are their impacts on the pelvic floor functions? **International Journal of Urology**, v. 39, n. 1, p. 46-54, 2013.

OLIVEIRA, M. M. F., *et al*. Manual lymphatic drainage and active exercises effects on lymphatic function do not translate into morbidities in women who underwent breast cancer surgery. **Arch. Phys. Med. Rehabil.**, v. 98, n. 2, p. 256-263, 2016.

ONG, T. A., et al. Using the Vibrance Kegel Device With Pelvic Floor Muscle Exercise for Stress Urinary Incontinence: A Randomized Controlled Pilot Study. **Urology**, v. 86, n. 3, p. 487-491, 2015.

OSANN, K., et al. Factors Associated with Poor Quality of Life among Cervical Cancer Survivors: Implications for Clinical Care and Clinical Trials. **Journal Gynecologic Oncology**, n. 135, n. 2, p. 266-272, 2014.

OZENGIN, N., et al. The effect of pelvic organ prolapse type on sexual function, muscle strength, and pelvic floor symptoms in women: A retrospective study. **Turk J. Obstet. Gynecol.**, v. 14, p. 121-127, 2017.

OZENGIN, O.; YILDIRIM, N. U.; DURAN, B. A comparison between stabilization exercises and pelvic floor muscle training in women with pelvic organ prolapse. **J. Turk Soc Obstet Gynecol.**, v. 1, p. 11-17, 2015.

PACIK, D.; FEDORKO, M. Literature review of factors affecting continence after radical prostatectomy. **Saudi Med. J.**, v. 38, n. 1, p. 9-17, 2017.

PAKBAZ, M.; ROLFSMAN, E.; LOFGREN, M. Are women adequately informed before gynaecological surgery? **BMC Women's Health**, v. 17, n. 68, p. 1-5, 2017.

PARK, J. H. The effects of complex exercise on shoulder range of motion and pain for women with breast cancer-related lymphedema: a single-blind, randomized controlled trial. **Breast Cancer**, v. XX, n. XX, p. 1-7, 2016.

PARK, J. W., et al. Predictors of adverse pathologic features after radical prostatectomy in low-risk prostate cancer. **BMC Cancer**, v. 18, n. 545, p. 1-7, 2018.

PARSA, Y., *et al*. A review of the clinical implications of breast cancer biology. **Electronic Physician**, v. 8, n. 5, p. 2416-2424, 2016.

PEDRAZA, R., et al. Pelvic muscle rehabilitation: a standardized protocol for pelvic floor dysfunction. **Advances in Urology**, v. 2014, p. 1-7, 2014.

PEREZ, F. S. B., et al. Effects of biofeedback in preventing urinary incontinence and erectile dysfunction after radical prostatectomy. **Front. Oncol.**, v. 8, n. 20, p. 1-20, 2018.

PÉREZ-SOLIS, A. M., et al. Effects of the lifestyle habits in breast cancer transcriptional regulation. **Cancer Cell Int.**, v. 16, n. 7, p. 1-11, 2016.

PETRILLO, M., et al. State of the art of prostatic arterial embolization for benign prostatic hyperplasia. **Gland. Surg.**, v. 7, n. 2, p. 188-199, 2018.

PLESCA, M., *et al*. Evolution of radical mastectomy for breast cancer. **J. Med. Life**, v. 9, n. 2, p. 183-

186, 2016.

PROVENCHER, L., *et al.* Is clinical breast examination important for breast cancer detection? **Curr. Oncol.**, v. 23, n. 4, p. 332-339, 2016.

QUIN, T., *et al.* Efficacy and tolerability of toremifene and tamoxifen therapy in premenopausal patients with operable breast cancer: a retrospective analysis. **Curr. Oncol.**, v. 20, n. 4, p. 196-204, 2013.

RAJKOWSKA-LABON, E., et al. Efficacy of Physiotherapy for Urinary Incontinence following Prostate Cancer Surgery. **BioMed Research International**, v. 2014, p. 1-9, 2014.

RIEF, W., *et al.* Long-term course of pain in breast cancer survivors: A four-year longitudinal study. **Breast Cancer Res. Treat.**, v. 130, n. 2, p. 579-586, 2011.

ROH, J. W., et al. Efficacy and oncologic safety of nerve-sparing radical hysterectomy for cervical cancer: a randomized controlled trial. **Journal Gynecologic Oncology**, v. 26, n. 2, p. 90-9, 2015.

SALLAMI, S. Predictive factors of urinary incontinence after radical prostatectomy: a systematic review. **Tunisia Mèdica**, v. 95, n. 4, 2017.

SALMON, V. E., et al. Opportunities, challenges and concerns for the implementation and uptake of pelvic floor muscle assessment and exercises during the childbearing years: protocol for a critical interpretive synthesis. **Systematic Reviews**, v. 6, n. 18, p. 19, 2017.

SAMUEL, S. R., *et al.* Exercise-based interventions for cancer survivors in India: a systematic review. **Springer Plus**, v. 4, n. 655, p. 1-16, 2015.

SANTOS, N. A. S., et al. Assessment of Physical Therapy Strategies for Recovery of Urinary Continence after Prostatectomy. **Asian Pac J Cancer Prev.**, v. 18, n. 1, p. 81-86, 2018.

SARTORI, D. V. B., et al. Reliability of pelvic floor muscle strength assessment in healthy continent women. **BMC Urology,** v. 15, n. 29, p. 1-6, 2015.

SATHIANATHEN, N. J., et al. The phytological future of prostate cancer staging: PSMA- PET and the dandelion theory. **Future Oncol.**, v. 13, n. 20, p. 1801-1807, 2017.

SCHMITT, J. J., et al. Prospective Outcomes of a Pelvic Floor Rehabilitation Program Including Vaginal Electrogalvanic Stimulation for Urinary, Defecatory, and Pelvic Pain Symptoms. **Female Pelvic Med Reconstr Surg**, v. 23, n. 2, p.108-113, 2017.

SEHL, M., *et al.* Decline in physical functioning in first 2 years after breast cancer diagnosis predicts

10-year survival in older women. **J. Cancer Surviv.**, v. 7, n. 1, p. 1-22, 2013.

SILVA, A. P. M., et al. Perineal Massage Improves the Dyspareunia Caused by Tenderness of the Pelvic Floor Muscles. **Rev. Bras. Gynecol. Obstet.**, v. 39, p. 26-30, 2017.

SMEETS, A., *et al*. Is the sentinel lymph node biopsy more sensitive for the identification of positive lymph nodes in breast cancer than the axillary lymph node dissection? **SpringerPlus**, v. 2, n. 275, p. 1-5, 2013.

STEIN, R. G., *et al*. The impact of breast cancer biological subtyping on tumor size assessment by ultrasound and mammography - a retrospective multicenter cohort study of 6543 primary breast cancer patients. **B. M. C. Cancer,** v. 16, n. 459, p. 1-8, 2016.

STOUT, N. L., *et al*. A prospective surveillance model for rehabilitation for women with breast cancer. **Cancer**, v. 118, n. 8, p. 2191-200, 2012.

SUN, X. L., et al. Effect of transcutaneous electrical stimulation treatment on lower urinary tract symptoms after class III radical hysterectomy in cervical cancer patients: study protocol for a multicentre, randomized controlled trial. **BMC Cancer**, v. 17, n. 416, p. 1-7, 2017.

TADA, H., et al. Risk factors for lower limb lymphedema after lymph node dissection in patients with ovarian and uterine carcinoma. **BMC Cancer**, v. 9, n. 47, p. 1-6, 2009.

TAJALI, S. M., *et al*. Reliability and Validity of Electro-Goniometric Range of Motion Measurements in Patients with Hand and Wrist Limitations. **Open Orthop. J.**, v. 10, p. 190-205, 2016.

TAMBOUR, M., *et al*. Effect of physical therapy on breast cancer related lymphedema: protocol for a multicenter, randomized, single-blind, equivalence trial. **B. M. C. Cancer J.,** v. 14, n. 239, p. 1-6, 2014.

TEHRANI, A. M., *et al*. Belonging to a peer support group enhance the quality of life and adherence rate in patients affected by breast cancer: a non-randomized controlled clinical trial. **J. Res. Med. Sci.**, v. 16, n. 5, p. 658-665, 2011.

TORRE, S.; MILLER, L. E. Multimodal vaginal toning for bladder symptoms and quality of life in stress urinary incontinence. **Int. Urogynecol. J.**, v. 2017, n. 28, p. 1201-1207, 2017.

TOSUN, O. C., et al. Assessment of the effect of pelvic floor exercises on pelvic floor muscle strength using ultrasonography in patients with urinary incontinence: a prospective randomized controlled trial. **J. Phys. Ther. Sci.**, v. 28, n. 2, p. 360-365, 2016.

TOVAR, J. R.; ZANDONADE, E.; AMORIM, M. H. Factors associated with the incidence of local recurrences of breast cancer in women who underwent conservative surgery. **Int. J. Breast Cancer,** v. 2014, p. 1-9, 2014.

URH, A., et al. Postoperative outcomes after continent versus incontinent urinary diversion at the time of pelvic exenteration for gynecologic malignancies. **Gynecologic Oncology**, v. 129, n. 3, p. 580-585, 2013.

URQUHART, D. M., et al. Regional morphology of the transversus abdominis and obliquus internus and externus abdominis muscles. **Clinical Biomechanics,** v. 20, p. 233241, 2005.

VILSBOLL, A. W., et al. Cell-based therapy for the treatment of female stress urinary incontinence: an early cost-effectiveness analysis. **Regen.Med.**, v. 13, n. 3, p. 321-330, 2018.

VOLLOYHAUG, I., et al. Assessment of pelvic floor muscle contraction with palpation, perineometry and transperineal ultrasound: a cross-sectional study. **Ultrasound Obstet Gynecol.**, v. 47, p. 768-773, 2016.

WANG, W., et al. Effectiveness of preoperative pelvic floor muscle training for urinary incontinence after radical prostatectomy: a meta-analysis. **BMC Urology**, v. 14, n. 99, p. 1-8, 2014.

WARE, R. A.; NAGELL, V. J. Radical Hysterectomy with Pelvic Lymphadenectomy: Indications, Technique, and Complications. **Obstetrics and Gynecology International,** v. 2010, p. 587-610, 2010.

WENWEN, W., et al. Evaluation of pelvic visceral functions after modified nerve-sparing radical hysterectomy. **Chinese Medical Journal**, v. 127, n. 4, p. 696-701, 2014.

WILSON, D. J. Exercise for the patient after breast cancer surgery. **Semin. Oncol. Nurs.**, v. XX, n. XX, p. 1-8, 2017.

WONG, A.; NGEOW, J. Hereditary Syndromes Manifesting as Endometrial Carcinoma: How Can Pathological Features Aid Risk Assessment? **BioMed Research International**, v. 2015, p. 1-17, 2015.

XU, M., et al. ErbB2 and p38γ MAPK mediate alcoholinduced increase in breast cancer stem cells and metastasis. **Molecular Cancer**, v. 15, n. 52, p. 1-14, 2016.

YAKOUB, D., *et al.* Factors associated with contralateral preventive mastectomy. **Breast Cancer (Auckl),** v. 2015, n. 7, p. 1-8, 2015.

YAMADA, Y., et al. Treatment strategy for metastatic prostate cancer with extremely high PSA level: reconsidering the value of vintage therapy. Asian Journal of Andrology, v. 20, p. 1-6, 2018.

YEN, T. W. F., *et al.* The interplay between hospital and surgeon factors and the use of sentinel lymph node biopsy for breast cancer. **Medicine,** v. 95, n. 31, p. 1-9, 2016.

YI, W. M., et al. Acupuncture for Preventing Complications after Radical Hysterectomy: A Randomized Controlled Clinical Trial. **Evidence-Based Complementary and Alternative Medicine**, v. 2014, p. 1-6, 2014.

YUNFENG, G., et al. Exercise overcomes adverse effects among prostate cancer patients receiving androgen deprivation therapy. **Medicine**, v. 96, n. 27, p. 1-10, 2017.

ZARSKI, A. C.; BERKING, M.; EBERT, D. D. Efficacy of Internet-Based Guided treatment for Genito-Pelvic Pain/Penetration Disorder: rationale, treatment Protocol, and Design of a randomized controlled trial. **Frontiers in Psychiatry**, v. 8, n. 260, p. 1-12, 2018.

ZHANG, M., et al. Risk prediction model for epithelial ovarian cancer using molecular markers and clinical characteristics. **Journal of Ovarian Research**, v. 8, n. 67, p. 1-12, 2015.

ZHANG, Y., *et al.* The 36-Item Short Form Health Survey: reliability and validity in Chinese medical students. **Int. J. Med. Sci.**, v. 9, n. 7, p. :521-526, 2012.

ZHOU, Y., et al. Prognostic value of circulating tumor cells in ovarian cancer: A MetaAnalysis. **PlosOne**, v. 10, n. 6, p. 1-14, 2015.

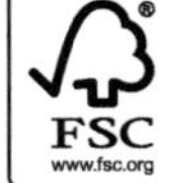

MIX
Papier aus verantwortungsvollen Quellen
Paper from responsible sources
FSC® C105338

Printed by Books on Demand GmbH, Norderstedt / Germany